HEAL YOUR LIFE

WITH

HOME REMEDIES

AND

HERBS

Other Books by Hanna Kroeger

❋

*Ageless Remedies from Mother's Kitchen
Allergy Baking Recipes
Alzheimer's Science and God
Arteriosclerosis and Herbal Chelation
Cancer: Traditional and New Concepts
Cookbook for Electro-Chemical Energies
God Helps Those Who Help Themselves
Good Health Through Special Diets
Hanna's Workshop
Healing with Herbs and Home Remedies A–Z
How to Counteract Environmental Poisons
*Instant Herbal Locator
*Instant Vitamin-Mineral Locator
*New Book on Healing
*New Dimensions in Healing Yourself
*Old-time Remedies for Modern Ailments
Parasites: The Enemy Within
The Pendulum, the Bible and Your Survival
The Seven Spiritual Causes of Ill Health
*Spices to the Rescue

❋

*The works indicated by an asterisk
have been combined for this book.

Please visit the Hay House Website at:
www.hayhouse.com

HEAL YOUR LIFE

WITH

HOME REMEDIES

AND

HERBS

Hanna Kroeger

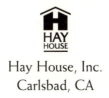

Hay House, Inc.
Carlsbad, CA

Copyright © 1998 by Hanna Kroeger

Published and distributed in the United States by:
Hay House, Inc., P.O. Box 5100, Carlsbad, CA 92018-5100
(800) 654-5126 • (800) 650-5115 (fax)

Edited by: Gretchen Lalik of Kroeger Herb Products;
           and Dee Bakker and Jill Kramer of Hay House

Designed by: Highpoint Graphics

Library of Congress Cataloging-in-Publication Data

Kroeger, Hanna.
    Heal your life with home remedies and herbs / by Hanna Kroeger.
         p.   cm.
    ISBN 1-56170-512-8
    1. Herbs—Therapeutic use.   2. Naturopathy.   Healing.   I. Title.
RM666.H33K76   1998
615'.321—dc21

                                                              97-50148
                                                              CIP

ISBN 1-56170-512-8

02 01 00 99   6 5 4 3
First Printing, April 1998
Third Printing, April 1999

Printed in the United States of America

CONTENTS

INTRODUCTION

This book is an accumulation of a lifetime of research and is intended to give you some real confidence and practical information on healing and show you how you can truly help yourself and others. Our understanding of healing is growing and changing. For instance, we used to lay all responsibility for our healing on the physicians, the priests, or the medicine men. Not any longer. Now we recognize that it is greatly our individual responsibility to stay well and to search every avenue to be healed. We need to be our own detectives. The use of all others outside ourselves should be but a support system for our learning. Included are our physicians, chiropractors, nutritionists, and those who show us spiritual and mental energies that lie unused and dormant in the depths of our being.

Knowledge of our spiritual and our physical selves coupled with an understanding of the amazing therapeutic values in foods and herbs will allow us to take an active role in healing ourselves and our families. Food and spices have always been an important part of life. Today, even with the hundreds and hundreds of drugs on the market, we still go to the kitchen and prepare specific food for the sick. We still apply liniments and compresses and concoct teas out of spices and herbs. We continue to do this because the old remedies and recipes work without danger of poisoning the system, and because we instinctively recognize that we must return to nature to heal ourselves. Remember, in no way will good, natural, nonchemical, or unadulterated food and a cup of good herbal tea interfere with our physician's work. Our physician will be happy that we are more balanced—that we have more strength and endurance to weather long-term illnesses.

I have decided to start this book with a discussion of our spiritual, mental, and physical characteristics and how they impact our overall health. This is followed by a section on diet and fasting. The final section includes a table of health issues and corresponding home remedies, a list of herb types, and recipes for oils and tinctures. This book is your guide for healing, and the tools are within you and your kitchen. In order to take full advantage of the healing power that lies within each one of us, we have to cooperate with nature and allow God's miracle foods and herbs to do their work.

Part I

---❊---

HEALING OUR SPIRITUAL, MENTAL, AND PHYSICAL SELVES

Chapter One

❋

SOUL LEVEL

It is important to remember that no illness ever resulted from a single cause. There are always several causes present. It stands to reason then that there is not a single method of healing therapy. Best results in healing come from a combination of therapies. Balancing our aura and its energy centers is one aspect of healing. It's vital that we understand how our negative traits directly influence our aura and our physical body.

For example, problems of the soul level can be expressed in the following physical natures:

- Heart trouble
- Low blood pressure
- High blood pressure
- Emotional troubles
- Paralyzed condition in parts or total
- Cramps
- Rheumatism
- Mental illness
- Mental limitations

In order to help, we have to bring our body and spirit into balance. Most probably you have heard the word *chakra*. This word is taken from Eastern philosophy, and it means *energy center*.

Eastern philosophy teaches that there are seven chakras in the human body. These teachings are better utilized once we understand that Eastern, Western, and Native American bodies have different energy centers. The Western body has two additional chakras or energy centers, and the Native American body has one additional chakra or energy center.

The Eastern Method

1. Base chakra (Kundalini)
2. Sacral chakra
3. Solar plexus chakra
4. Heart chakra
5. Throat chakra
6. Forehead chakra (pituitary)
7. Crown chakra (pineal)

The Easterner recognizes that these seven chakras are brought into balance by:

- Lotus position (sitting cross-legged)
- Mantra repetition
- Meditation
- Incense

The Easterner may sit under a mango tree meditating all day to attain the highest balance. The Westerner and the Native American would not likely attain the highest balance using this method.

The Native American Method

The Native American has eight chakras, the additional chakra being located at the sacrum, accessed from the back. This is where he takes in his energy. The Native American brings the chakras into balance by:

- Sweat baths
- Circle dances
- Sage incense
- Drumming

The Native American will use rituals to connect with the Creator.

The Western Method

The Westerner has nine chakras:

1. Light chakra (light enters at the seventh cervical vertebra, accessed from the back)
2. Action chakra (allows us to put ideas into action; located at the base, accessed from the back)
3. Base chakra (Kundalini)
4. Sacral chakra (reproductive, bowels)
5. Solar plexus chakra (seat of emotional body)
6. Heart chakra
7. Throat chakra (will)
8. Forehead chakra (pituitary)
9. Crown chakra (pineal)

The Westerner's methods to bring the light centers, or chakras, to work are:

- Prayer
- Singing
- Action
- Visualization
- Contemplation

The Westerner is more apt to get his visions and intuitive guidance by moving the body—taking a long walk, jogging, hiking, shoveling snow, driving a tractor, moving hay bales, or even singing.

The colors of the Westerner's nine light centers are:

1. Red
2. Orange

3. Yellow
4. Green
5. Blue
6. Magenta
7. Violet
8. Pink
9. White

We can use either of the following two methods to bring our light centers into balance.

FIRST METHOD

Visualize the centers with the respective colors and balance them by visualization. This takes about ten minutes total.

SECOND METHOD

Intake and output have to be alike. So, fold your hands and make a triangle over the seventh vertebra. Ask loudly for the color red, the universal power, the color of strength, for 30 seconds. Then place your hand above the head, going up and down, saying "intake and output have to be alike." Do this for 30 seconds, and the miracle is that all centers are aligned, all at once.

Synchronizing Your Brain

After you have balanced your light centers, synchronize your brain. Your brain is your control tower. It has to be in balance. Take a crystal in your left hand. The crystal should not be cut, one side being rough. A crystal is a tool that multiplies your thoughts many times.

Talk to the crystal: "I will that you become an instrument of our Lord, that you help to balance this person's brain."

Now picture the five sections of the brain by envisioning the scalp (on the top of your head). Beginning with the back left portion is Section I; Section II is the front left; Section III is the back right; Section IV is front right; and Section V is the center portion. Take each section of the brain and say, "In the name of the Most High, be balanced!" Go from section to section. Every time, ask for balance. Now you are in balance. Now you are ready to heal others. Give thanks to our Lord.

How do you know when your brain is out of balance? When one shoulder is higher than the other. When one leg is shorter than the other. When the right eye droops. When the jaw is misaligned.

Hold your hands together. One hand will be longer. Synchronize the brain and all that comes into balance.

Prayer Action Plan for Dissolving the Spiritual Cause of a Physical Problem

Hawaiian Kahunas used to get rid of unwanted negative attitudes and feelings by relaxing and commanding these unwanted negative attitudes to leave their bodies while they shook their right and left legs.

I suggest taking the following steps:

1. Review the situation that is presently causing a particular emotional stress.

2. Pick a word that expresses the positive opposite of this negative emotion. (For example: You hate—think of love. You are anxious—think of security. You worry—think of confidence, etc.)

3. Place a glass of water next to you.

4. Relax. See yourself beset with the negative emotion. Put it all into the glass of water. Throw the water away.

5. Take a fresh cup, preferably porcelain. Fill this cup with water, and think that this water contains the necessary solution to your problem—it is filled with the opposite, positive emotion. Drink the water, knowing that you are filling yourself with the positive emotion you need. The negativity will leave you when you next urinate.

6. End session. Then urinate, feeling an exhilaration of positivity.

Chapter Two

MIND AND BODY CONNECTION

"To think is the hardest work there is. This is most probably the reason why so few people engage in it."
— Henry Ford

It is often said that man is the result of his environmental forces. This is not true. We cannot believe this, because the facts always prove the contrary. Many of the world's greatest men have been born in poverty and in adverse conditions.

Many who have been born in slums and filthy surroundings have risen to the highest status in the world. They have won laurels of fame and distinguished themselves in politics, literature, and poetry. They have become beacons of light in the world. How do we account for this?

Thought is the greatest force on earth. Thought is the most powerful weapon in the armor of a saint. Constructive thought transforms, renews, and builds. The far-reaching possibilities of this force were most accurately developed to perfection by the ancients and put to the highest possible use. Thought is the primal force at the origin of all creation; the genesis of the entire phenomenal creation is given as a single thought that arose in the cosmic mind.

However, the forces of thought, which are wireless messages, have to have an impulse. This impulse is found in the mitro-genetic rays. These are rays that appear for the first time in the brain. It has been found that when the frontal lobes of the brain are closer together, more of the mitro-genetic rays are released. We know that mitro-genetic rays differ in both quality and quantity. We know that by stimulating the frontal lobes, thoughts become streamlined and powerful.

The following method is terrific to streamline and give spark to your thoughts:

1. Massage your forehead with fingertips of each hand for 30 seconds.
2. Touch the spots on the back of your head just behind each ear. Hold for 30 seconds.
3. Touch the spot just below your right knee on the right side of the leg. Hold for 30 seconds.

The mitro-genetic ray is the real transporter of a thought. Without this ray, a thought is a bird without wings. The mitro-genetic ray gives the spark needed so that thoughts become reality. Natural healers are all born with a powerful mitro-genetic ray. We have to stimulate this ray to become self-healers.

Thoughts Can Promote Radiant Health

The body is internally associated with the mind; that is, the body is a counterpart of the mind. It is a gross, visible form of the subtle, invisible mind. If there is pain in the tooth or in the stomach or in the ear, the mind is at once affected. It ceases to think properly; it is agitated, disturbed, and perturbed.

Congestion of the mind can express itself in the physical realm as the following:

- Heart trouble
- Low blood pressure
- High blood pressure
- Emotional trouble
- Paralyzed condition in parts or total
- Cramps

- Rheumatism
- Mental illnesses
- Mental limitations
- Accidents
- Bone trouble
- Leukemia
- Stiff joints
- Deafness
- Congestion in digestive tracts

If we entertain negative thoughts of hate, envy, jealousy, or fear, we invite dark brothers and energies of darkness. If you have such unproductive thoughts, stand in front of your mirror and say loudly, "Stop, stop, stop!" and all the dark brothers leave, making room for angels. If we have happy and constructive thoughts, energy will follow them and build a healthy body and a happy environment.

Napoleon controlled his thoughts in this manner: "When I want to think of things more pleasant, I close the cupboards of my mind revealing the more unpleasant things of life, and open up the cupboards containing the more pleasant thoughts. If I want to sleep, I close up all the cupboards of mind!"

If the spoken word has to have power, it has to have enthusiasm. The sound of the spoken word affects the thyroid gland, then the thymus gland and the spleen. The thyroid, thymus, and spleen are the center of the immune system. Therefore, the spoken word is a constructive rebuilder.

The wave of the spoken word goes on in the pineal gland, stimulating it; then to the pituitary gland, balancing it; then on to the saliva glands, the solar plexus, and the adrenal glands. Every center in our body is affected by our speech. It intensifies or dissipates our aura.

The power of the spoken word is not only for ourselves, it is also for others. Every time we speak, we send out sounds through our etheric, astral, and mental centers. This is the mechanical way a spoken word goes. On its way to the aura, it stimulates or depresses all glands. The spoken word uplifts or destroys.

Acquisition of Thought Power by Moral Purity

A man who speaks the truth and has moral purity always has powerful thoughts. One who has controlled anger by long practice has tremendous thought power.

Thought Power by Concentration

There is no limit to the power of human thought. The more concentrated the human mind is, the more power is brought to bear on one point. Cultivate attention, and you will have good concentration. A serene mind is fit for concentration. Keep the mind serene, be cheerful always, and then you can concentrate. Be regular in your concentration. Always sit in the same place, at the same time.

Attaining Mental Clarity

To stimulate mental clarity, place your left hand on the left shoulder of your partner. Start at the bottom with one finger on each side of the spine and slowly move up. When you arrive at the point between the spine and the shoulder blades, draw your right hand under the left hand, and move both hands down over the arms. Shake your hands and start again. Do this several times.

Increasing Intelligence

This will help increase intelligence. Press thumbs on both temples, and at the same time, take a deep, slow breath. Then press the thumb of the left hand on the middle of forehead above and between the eyes and press the thumb of the right hand on the outside corner of the right eye. Take another deep breath, hold the mouth tight, and puff out the cheeks.

Chapter Three

HEALING HANDS

"The human hand is the antenna of the mind."

The hands are tools that the mind depends upon when it wants to get anything done. The laying on of hands has a wide range of meanings. The priests of old and the priests of today consecrated the laying on of hands, which means laying on the "Hands of God." It is a very holy act in our churches. Ministers are ordained by the laying on of hands. Special gifts are conferred to individuals with the laying on of hands.

The human hand is the antenna of the mind. It is the hand that conveys the healing thought of the healer to the sick person. By this method, healing vibrations are picked up by the tissue, nerves, and cells, and they quickly transfer the imprinted thought of health to other parts of the body.

If you have a telephone but do not speak into the speaker, the message will not be heard on the other end of the line. If you have a sick fellow man but you do not transfer your healing power of the hands through special "speaker places" on the body, the sick body cannot respond and cannot take the message.

The natural power, this healing element, is not limited to clergymen or priests. Nature gave mothers an unselfish readiness to help their offspring.

They place their hand on the feverish forehead, and they bathe the little bodies. They embrace the hurting, crying youngster.

You Can Heal

We all can heal—mainly ourselves. We all can help others to heal themselves. Doctors, practitioners, pharmacists, surgeons, and healers can only give the supply needed so that you can become whole.

To become whole, to be healed, is the work of the individual in need. Just as every art requires knowledge and practice, so does this art of healing require knowledge and practice. When you go to a painting or wood-carving class, you are instructed about the materials you'll use, such as paint, canvas, wood, and chisels. Whatever you create thereafter, it is the creative spirit in you that forms it, and you have the privilege through knowledge and practice to use your hands for creating new things and making old things new.

Pneumonia

The laying on of hands in pneumonia cases is the greatest joy that one can experience. Rest your right hand over the forehead of the one to whom you want to give energies, so that your finger rests on the middle of the nose. The left hand has to be placed on the back of the head so you really cradle the head (the right hand in the front, the left hand in the back). In this position, wait for 20 minutes. After ten minutes, you hear it cracking and working in the chest. After 20 minutes, the afflicted one will breathe freely. Then place your right hand over the chest bone, fingers facing toward the chin, the left hand on the back, and let more energies flow through for about five more minutes. Repeat as often as you think it is needed. Usually one time is all it takes. With babies, do it as soon as the first signs of a chest cold appear. Hold the baby in your lap and cradle its head.

Asthma

Let the child or adult suffering from asthma lie on the floor. Bend the knees and elevate them on a chair. Hands should brush stomach from midsection right and left under the rib cage. Do this over and over, ten minutes in the mornings and ten minutes in the evenings.

One teaspoon of cranberry concentrate opens the bronchi.

Ear Stimulation

This method will greatly assist in inner ear troubles and will also help in maintaining the balance.

The patient should lie on his back. The healer stands on the right side of patient and places the fingertips and thumb of his right hand into the patient's right hand. The fingertips of the healer's left hand are placed on a point at the base of the skull just below the right ear. Hold the hands for 30 seconds to help energy flow.

The healer then moves over to the left side of the patient and places the fingertips and thumb of his left hand into the patient's left hand. The fingertips of the healer's right hand are placed on a point at the base of the skull just below the right ear to complete the circuit. This is to be held for 30 seconds.

Stomach

This is good for underweight children and adults. Let the middle finger of your left hand rest in the "cup"—the bones in front of the throat. Place the right hand over the stomach. Do not place it flat, but form a cup out of your hand. Keep this hollow hand for 60 seconds, and then make small, soft semicircles over the stomach.

Do this once daily for seven days, then two times a week.

Kidney

The right kidney is positive magnetic in nature. Therefore, you have to place your left hand over the right kidney. The left kidney has a negative charge so your right hand has to be placed over the left kidney. Have your friend lie on his stomach. Stand to the side of his head and let your hands rest on his kidney as previously indicated.

Leave your hands resting for two to three minutes, then slowly rotate them in an open-loop manner toward the spine.

The touch must be very light and should last only for about one minute. Finally, give the nerves on the spine a little twisting motion. For this you touch a little firmer and in a round circular motion. Let them know that they have to start working again. Just after repairing your wiring in the house you turn on the switch. It is the same thing here.

Itching of Skin

When people itch all over, the following treatment is of great value. Brush body from head to toe with your hands spread out and thumbs touching each other.

- Front 7 times
- Back 7 times
- Right arm 7 times
- Left arm 7 times

Also hold the right hand over the left shoulder. Brush with the left hand the gallbladder and liver area.

Bed-Wetting

Behind the ears are two tiny holes. Massage these holes with a very light pressure. At the same time ask someone to rub the feet with a towel until they are warm.

Blood Clots

Make your friend comfortable on a bed or worktable. Flex his knees. Have his hands folded as in prayer, but his fingers should form a pyramid. His thumbs close it. Cover your friend with a light blanket for warmth and comfort. There is nothing like a blanket pulled over you that gives more security. Now sit on his left side. Spread your arms out so the right hand is close to the top of his head. The left hand is slipped under the cover. Hold it close to the tailbone. You cuddle your friend visibly and invisibly. Your hands do not touch the body at all, but are one inch away from it.

(The credit for this method goes to Rev. Dr. Fred M. Houston.)

Dropped Organs

For dropped organs, lie on your back. Hold right or left point of the cup on the collarbone while you lightly sweep up the body (pray in Jesus' name that the organs move up). Then do the same for the left side, then do the middle. Sweep up until the pain is gone. When finished, suture by holding the ankles until your hand feels the pulse.

Ovaries

See chapter 5 (Key Positions: Ovaries) for instructions.

Nervous Breakdown

Many people with nervous disorders have fallen arches. I notice that in many cases of insecure walking people have fallen arches. The following work will help to bring fallen arches back to normal position, and clearer thinking is the result. To bring arches back, apply pressure on the center peritoneal group of muscles.

Applied to people with a nervous breakdown, it works like a charm. In all these severe cases, you have to hold this key position until it gurgles three times. Just before it gurgles, these people start asking for release of the pressure applied. Do not give in. Wait until it gurgles or snaps under your fingers. The pressure is firm but not torturing, not a light touch. It will take up to 20 minutes for the third release. Some folks start crying. Put a lavender colored cloth over their face so no one sees the tears and agony when the old pattern is released.

Folks who have had a nervous breakdown years ago also have to be released. And what a release it is for them! In some cases it is needed to "soften" the keyhole to the emotional body first. Apply lavender oil or eucalyptus oil on the keyholes under the knees and one inch below the sternum. Lavender oil is the best.

Heart

To calm down a rapid heartbeat, hold the right hand over the head. Touch the middle of the head with one finger. Hold the left hand over the thyroid (wrap around neck). When you are emotionally troubled and you cannot sleep, try this method. It will calm you down, and relaxing sleep can come.

Hold spread fingers, palms facing forward and thumbs down, lightly against the sides of the face. It relaxes the heart muscle, which is very important in heart attacks.

The spoken word influences the heart chamber—it opens or closes it. It gives life power to the heart chamber, or it makes it malfunction. If in shock by bad news, by a harsh judgment, or by a word of fear, the heart chamber goes into spasms, and it can be so strong, so powerful, that people faint, pass out, or have a heart attack if conditions in the arteries are not right.

Take an herbal combination of hawthorn berries, *Equisetum* concentrate, vitamin C, taurine, arginine, chromium picolinate, and selenium. Aloe vera gel is also recommended.

Circulation

To stimulate circulation, place the left hand on top of the stomach, fingers pointing down. With your right hand, stroke the left leg with parallel strokes from the groin down over the left leg and foot. Interrupt the magnetic lock by shaking the hand and in a wide semicircle start at the groin and move down.

Eyes

This is used by American Indians: On the back of the head behind the ears are two little indentations. Hold these with both thumbs for one minute. The first thing you notice is that the protruding veins on the back of your hands get smaller. Hold and the protruding veins will vanish completely. It has a profound effect on the eyes and brings circulation to them. Second, gently, gently touch the outside corners of your eyes and massage toward the eyes. This relaxes tired eyes and will lubricate them.

Then, in case of cross-eyed condition, massage the middle of the ankle from the top. It has to be done very gently and twice every day.

Last, in case of pressure in the eyes, as in glaucoma, the points behind the jaw release the fluid in the eyes. These points have to be held ten minutes at a time, two times daily for three to four weeks. Hold both sides.

Diaphragm Area

This will help to give release to the rib cage on both sides and thus assist in energy breathing.

One will truly appreciate the relaxation this will produce on both sides of the chest area. It will also help to energize the gallbladder and the liver on the right side area and the spleen and pancreas on the left lower rib area.

Lie on your back. Put the palm of the right hand over the liver. Put the left hand on the neck area on the right side. Then place the left hand over the liver, and the right hand on the left side on neck.

General energy circulation will take place within the organs concerned.

How to use touch, pressure points, and hands to heal ourselves and others is described throughout the following chapters. These things may sound so simple, but effectiveness is what really matters.

Chapter Four

*

EMOTIONS

"When you know where you are going, the world steps aside."

D r. Candace Pert, Ph.D., chief of the institute section on Brain and Biochemistry at the National Institute of Mental Health in Bethesda, Maryland, stated, "Emotions are not just in the brain but are also in the body and appear to run the immune system, the glands, the intestines. So your whole body is a single-unit integrated circuit, running on biochemicals." Once all of this is fully understood, it may provide the medical profession with totally new ways to treat diseases such as cancer, schizophrenia, obesity, and AIDS.

Upset emotions can have visible manifestations in the following disease patterns:

- Toxic condition in lymph
- Toxic condition throughout the body
- Skin condition
- Hair loss
- Paralysis
- Metabolic disorders

We have two important glands for decongesting emotions. The first is the pineal gland. This is the master gland. It is located close to the pituitary gland, in the middle of the brain, a short distance behind the root of the nose. The pineal gland, when well developed, brings emotional and physical well-being. This gland is also the throne of our faith. As we develop faith, we develop the pineal gland. Faith alone has no power. So God gave us another gland right next to the pineal gland. It is the pituitary gland. The pituitary gland lies in the "Turkish saddle," well embedded, and it is the gland of imagination.

These two we may call twin glands. We can imagine that some kind of healing without the power of faith will not bring lasting results. On the other hand, faith—blind faith—without the goal of imagining, has no end result and will not open the doors for healing the body. For example, if someone is confined to a wheelchair or is bedridden, the first thing this person has to do—and with him all people concerned—is to imagine that he/she can walk again. And then believe what the mind sees. You cannot tell what comes first, imagining or faith. Both are needed for results. The first question is: How can we strengthen these mentioned glands, these powerhouses? The next question is: How can we line up these glands so they work together? In this chapter are some suggestions that have worked well for me and others.

The first gland affected by emotions is the thyroid gland, and with it, the parathyroid gland and then the thymus gland. Thyroid glands and thymus glands are part of the immune system. With the spoken word you influence your immune system right now.

It is known that in times of grief, people get viruses, the flu, and other infections. They say the cemetery was cold and windy, or in the chapel during the service, people were coughing and crying and spreading germs. The truth is that the power of the spoken word of sadness has depressed the immune system to an extent that people could not throw off the germs that were dormant in their system.

WHAT TO DO

An emotional crisis does more than injure your psyche. It jeopardizes your physical health. It increases your risk of sickness, and it can add to accidental injuries.

How can that be? Under stress, the normal immune system defense can break down, resulting in greater readiness to disease. Colds, the flu, mononucleosis, and even leukemia can be triggered by an emotional crisis.

What to do? Don't be passive. We all go through difficult times. We feel helpless, hopeless, and overwhelmed. Take a positive approach. Try this: Close your left eye. With your right eye, look into a mirror and stare into your eye's image and say, "Flu, you are gone. Get out of me, right now." Repeat several times. You will be amazed!

Problems always come in pairs or clusters. I make a list of the problem or problems I am confronted with. After writing them down, I read each one. I think them over, and I cut out the problem that can be solved the easiest. Then I go to the next one, and down the list, until I find one or two at the core, so to speak, at the center of the stress.

By unwrapping the problems in this manner, one can intelligently and almost totally solve the emotional stress that can make you sick.

Nervous Disorders

Many people with nervous disorders have fallen arches. I notice that many cases involving insecure walking are accompanied by fallen arches. The following work will help to bring fallen arches back to normal position, and clearer thinking is the result. To bring arches back, apply pressure on the center peroneal group of leg muscles (located near the fibula, the outer bone of the lower leg).

The Importance of Dealing with Emotions

How is it possible that feelings of anger, jealousy, hostility, and fear can affect our health? Are these feelings not just a passing situation? Unfortunately not, and I explain this with the following example.

When we are in a threatening situation, the stress hormones—adrenaline and its companion, noradrenaline—are poured out in great quantity. These hormones stimulate the brain to quick and immediate action. From there the excess reaches the arterial system and adds to the formation of plaque buildup. The cortex of the adrenal gland is stimulated by resentment, jealousy, or feelings of defeat, and it releases a hormone called cortisol. This would not be dangerous in small doses; however, prolonged resentments and affiliated feelings put out so much cortisol that your health is threatened from within.

Why is that? Cortisol is released by the cortex of the adrenal gland. Too much cortisol diminishes the power of the immune system by depressing the natural killer cells. Natural killer cells are watchdogs of the immune system and destroy dangerous and abnormal cells as needed. When too many abnormal, fungus-type cells take over, these fungus-type cells may develop into tumors.

Another bad thing about uncontrolled, prolonged emotions and emotional stress is that precious interferon cannot be manufactured, and T cells and B cells receive no nourishment.

We live in a stressful world. What can we do to stay emotionally sound?

- Examine the problem.
- Singing in groups in churches or by yourself reduces and releases emotional stress.
- Recite a poem.
- Physical exercises help tremendously.
- Look at a problem with a humorous outlook. In every problem is something funny.
- Believe in something sacred and holy or in things that stimulate happiness and thankfulness.

Grief

Whenever we lose a beloved one, naturally we grieve. However, some of us grieve so intensely that we cannot carry on with our lives. We go from physician to minister, from priest to friends, and they all say the same: "You will get over the loss in time."

The grieving person is blocked in life, and so is the aura of the parted one. Excessive, prolonged grief holds the aura of the parted one, keeping him in limbo. You have to let go. The following ceremony will help you.

Every day for 14 days (some of us need more time) perform the following ritual. Put a mat on the floor so that your head will be north. Light seven candles and place them in a wide circle around the mat. Light-colored candles such as pink, blue, or white are best. Now lie relaxed on the mat. Meditate and pray. After a while, talk to your beloved one in the following manner: "I release you. I love you. Because I love you, I will not grieve any longer, so you can be happy. Go on to your new task." Talk to your parted one and stay relaxed for 30 minutes and know that all is well. Repeat if needed.

Jealousy

Jealousy is one of the most destructive emotions a person can carry. It causes all kinds of physical ailments.

- Stomach trouble
- Aches and pains
- Indigestion
- Headaches
- Lung trouble
- Liver trouble

Jealousy is like a boil that is emptying its foul contents into your beautiful body. The following method helps most people overcome jealousy. Make a tea of the following:

- 2 oz. cyany flower
- 2 oz. chamomile
- 2 oz. rose petal
- 2 oz. orange blossom
- 2 oz. spearmint

Mix. Add 1 tsp. of this mixture to 1 cup of boiling water. Drink 1 cup. Then place the middle finger of your right hand 2 inches below your navel. Hold the middle finger of the left hand on the back of the skull. Say loudly, "I release the jealousy that I carry toward (say name or situation). I release this negative entity now, and I am free from a burden that made me sick and not fully productive. Jealousy stood in my way to Christ." It is released now.

We realize that jealousy is the root of hate, war, disease, resentment, and marriage trouble. It is worth fighting against this huge, destructive force. Jealousy is one big factor that holds you back from spiritual growth and spiritual advancement. It is like a magnet that draws all ills, pain, and fear to you. You have to make personal and sacrificial effort to release jealousy; then all other difficulties will be solved.

ANOTHER METHOD

Relax in a chair. Have a glass of water next to you. Pile up all difficulty and jealousy you might have toward a person or a situation and throw it into the water. After a few minutes, throw this water down the drain. Do not give it to a plant. The plant will wither. Now fill the cup with water and add 1 tsp. apple cider vinegar. Fill the water with the good thoughts of your inner self, then drink it. All jealousy is gone, and you start a new life. To release resentment, do the same thing.

Depression

Sometimes we suffer from depression, which we desire to overcome quickly. The following method is highly advisable. However, if your depression comes from low blood sugar syndrome, *Candida albicans*, or any other serious physical ailment, it will not help.

You have to use a lot of energy to keep yourself depressed. Frequently, depression is anger turned inward. If you let go, depression can be eliminated. Hold the following points: under the chin; at the base of the breastbone; the right side of the kneecap on the right leg; on the inner right side of the rib cage, about two inches below the base of the breastbone.

Fear and Depression

Hold the same points and, in addition, the right side below the floating rib, the inside of both elbows, and on the right middle finger. Fear and distrust with depression are always experienced when you do not breathe deeply and exhale fully. Put deep breathing on your program.

Lack of Self-Confidence

Lack of self-confidence can bring a person to highest performance, or it can toss his life into total misery. In severe cases, psychotherapy is needed. However, you could try the following method, which works quickly and is inexpensive.

Press behind both ears. You will find a bony indentation. Hold this for 30 seconds. Next, press the points (right and left) under the skull behind the head, for 30 seconds. In addition, press firmly in the middle of the soles of your feet for 30 seconds. Lastly, press on the heels (middle) from the bottom of your feet for 30 seconds. Do this every morning and every night.

Forgiveness

One of the greatest difficulties we have to overcome is forgiveness—forgiving ourselves and forgiving others. Serious illnesses carry a seed of unforgiving in the mind and heart, and it acts like acid, eating away at our health. Our Lord Jesus, suffering on the cross, said, "Father, forgive them." Forgiveness was so important to him that He mentioned it in His last hour.

The following method, given to us by Dr. Duane Anderson, is a tremendous help:

Imagine the top of your head divided into four equal sections. Then, stand straight with the middle finger of your right hand touching the left back portion of the scalp (on the top of your head) and with a rubbing motion, say, "In the name of our Lord, I forgive myself and I forgive (place, name). I forgive totally."

Next, with the middle finger of the right hand, touch the left front portion of the scalp (on top of your head) and say the same thing, with the same rubbing motion. Then, with the middle finger of the left hand on the right back portion of the scalp, say the same thing. Finally, with the middle finger of the left hand on the right front portion of the scalp, say the same again. Place your right hand above the navel and say, "I forgive myself; I forgive those who did me wrong." At the same time, rub around your navel seven times in a clockwise motion. A great relief will come over you.

Sorrow

Hold your hands over your heart. Cup your hands and visualize placing your heart into your hands. Slowly move your cupped hands forward, visualizing giving your heart to the Lord. Then offer the heart and your sorrow, love, and life to God.

Sadness

Sit down, cross your legs, with the right ankle resting on top of the left leg (left foot on the floor). Place your left hand just below the knee of your right leg, and with your right hand (crossing over the left arm), press on the instep of the right foot. Then reverse the position.

Anger

Anger can be a holy anger. Christ took his whip and cleared the temple of the cheating merchants. Anger can arouse a person to tremendous powers, as shown in these examples:

- A middle-aged woman saw two huge men molesting a young girl. The girl screamed, but no one paid attention—no one wanted to tangle with these men. The woman got so angry that she took her umbrella, opened it, and rammed it into one of the fellows. He fled and so did the other crook.

- One young man started a business. It looked as if it would fail. Neighbors and his relatives laughed and said, "You are a failure to begin with." He got so angry that, in spite of all the odds, he made it, and he made it big.

- Two fellows started a fist fight of a serious nature in front of my little store. The huge window pane started to quiver back and forth. I got so angry that I took a broom and beat them up with it, and so saved my window and stopped the fight.

When we can arouse cancer victims to anger about themselves and their situation, we have almost won the battle. Cancer victims need that holy sword of anger, and they are then able to heal themselves.

A person with paralysis does not need sympathy, he or she needs the holy sword of anger. It will knit the nerve connections. They have to do it for themselves, and they will succeed. By the way, take them out of the chair and let them crawl on their knees. Below the knees is the entrance to the central nervous system. When treated this way, it repairs itself. No wonder the churches had such results. They put their holy shrines way up on the mountains. Those seeking help had to crawl up on their knees. There were no cars or horse carriages, and, wonder over wonder, when they arrived, after hours or even days, their ailments were gone.

When anger is not released constructively, however, it turns into resentment. It can turn into violence; it can turn into destruction, particularly for the one who carries it. Anger can turn into hate. Hate is extremely destructive to the liver. The liver has to detoxify the chemicals, environmental poisons, metal poisons, and so on. If one is filled with hate, the liver cannot do its job, and the poison goes into the bloodstream, creating all kinds of trouble such as allergies, flu, hives, mood swings, and emotional upsets.

Releasing Anger and Resentment

Try the following methods to release anger and resentment:

1. Firmly stroke over your face and head with both hands. Start at your chin, slowly move up to your forehead, over your hair to the back of your head, and end at the neck. Repeat: chin, forehead, back of head, neck. Repeat several times. This will release resentments—even childhood resentments and hidden anger.

2. In the evening, write all your angers, resentments, or shortcomings on a piece of paper. Not an old piece of scratch paper, but a nice piece of paper, as if you were writing a letter to a dear friend. Do not read it. Put it in a drawer. The next morning, read it and burn it. In the evening, do it again. Do this until all resentment is gone— one week or three days—it depends on you. This is cheaper than

burdening a psychiatrist with your troubles. This will release pain, sore throat, and even cancer.

3. Sit on a chair and press your thumbs against the middle of your thighs. Say these words:

> Ah-Kai-Ion
> Ah is the color gold,
> Kai is the color blue,
> Ion is the color white.

This will remove unpleasant memory patterns of which resentments are a part.

Fear

Fear is an emotion that paralyzes. If I see a snake, I stand still from fear. If you are afraid, your T cells in the immune system freeze up. They stand still and close up, and your immune system goes way down.

I have an easy way to overcome fear, and you will laugh at it, but it works. Pinch your buttocks, pinch them hard, and all fear vanishes.

Love is an emotion. You may have self-love, or you may have the attribute of God that is true love, and this will open for you the doors of great happiness of light and healing.

WHAT TO DO

What can be done? How can we keep the connection between the thymus and heart open? Pound your breastbone for one or two minutes, and then start rolling your head. Do both pounding your breastbone and rolling your head at the same time for one more minute. Soon you will feel warmth coming to your heart, you'll start yawning or sighing (or both), and an unaccountable happiness will spread over you. The secretion of the thymus in an adult makes an etheric stream and increases intelligence, self-esteem, happiness, and trust. In addition, the herb thyme is very valuable in keeping the thymus gland in good shape.

Freeing Yourself

In May 1953, our family arrived as refugees in America. We brought along five children, several sacks of old clothes, some tools, and featherbeds all packed in a tin bathtub. I thought that we had to start out like the old settlers in the wilderness, and I wanted to be sure my children got a bath once a week. I did not know that America was so highly civilized.

Once we settled down, my husband, an engineer, found work, and I went housecleaning. Something was bothering me. Every night, night after night, I was reliving the past. The nights of terror, the bombing, the hopelessness, the uncertainty if my husband would return from captivity in Russia. I was exhausted in the morning. I felt my health slipping. My first cousin was a psychiatrist in Milwaukee, and I asked her what to do about it. She gave the following advice: "Take a paper and pen. Every night when you are alone, sit down and write out what you experienced. Don't read it over. Put the writing in a drawer. Next morning read it and burn it. Do this for a week or until you have nothing to report to yourself."

I started that very evening. After a week, I was free. I was free from the old stuff that was hindering me to start a new life. Every morning when I reread the written notes, it was like a fictional story.

I went back to my cousin and thanked her and asked, "Elizabeth, how did this work? Why did this work? I have tried so many things, but this worked."

She answered, "As you speak your troubles out, they become larger, bigger, tremendous, voluminous in size, but when you write it out, read it the next day, and burn it, it takes on a different dimension. It is out of your brain, it is out of every cell of your body, and you are free and can stay well."

Thank you forever, Elizabeth. I have given this formula to many, many troubled people, and every time it works. Free yourself from the old pattern, and you open yourself to new and better experiences. My health returned in one week, and so will yours. Try it.

This knowledge is particularly important after a painful divorce. Make yourself free from a terrible nightmare of guilt and start anew. It is often the case that when men and women remarry, they find themselves in the same situation that they left behind. Why is that so? It is because they did not free themselves. The way it was shown to me by a psychiatrist is the surest way to total success.

❧ ✿ ❧

Chapter Five

---✻---

KEY POSITIONS

Our bodies are composed of different systems. These systems have to work together. When one system is diseased, all systems suffer. When the blood is sick, the transportation of life force is interrupted. When the decalcification of the bones takes place, everything suffers. Each of these systems has a master key, a point by which the systems are influenced. Holding a point will influence a particular system. The key positions of the following systems are known.

Skeletal System

Hold the seventh cervical vertebra. Do not rub, do not manipulate, just hold. It will influence favorably and heal the entire system. If you have broken a bone, this point will be sore, but it also will heal any bone in the system when you hold it long enough. The rule is, hold this point for three days in a row (a friend may have to help hold for you), and your bone will be healed. For the elderly it will take six days to accomplish this.

COMFREY ROOT TINCTURE

This is a bone strengthener and helps with bone pain, broken bones, and stump pain. Take five drops in water. Also, place one drop on the seventh cervical vertebra.

Ligaments

The key position for the ligaments (all ligaments in the body) is a point above the elbow of your right arm. Open your hand. From the thumb upward, over the elbow and directly on the bone, you will find a sore spot. Hold it for 60 seconds. It will hurt when needed. You will feel the ligaments going into place wherever it was needed.

DANDELION ROOT TINCTURE

For injuries to muscles and tendons, make compresses and apply to point described above.

Muscles

The key position of all muscles in the body is just below the calves. Sit on a chair. Flex your knees and hold the point firmly until the pain is gone.

Lymphatic System

The lymphatic system becomes sluggish with a lack of exercise. In all cases of cancer, the lymphatic system should be stimulated. Do not implement Swedish massage. In cancer patients it is too dangerous because cancer is easily transferred from one place to another. By stimulating the following points, the lymph will carry out trapped garbage and protein. See also chapter 6 (Glands: Lymph Gland [Node]).

The key position for the lymphatic system is with the right hand placed in the left armpit, and the left hand held over the seventh cervical vertebra. The fingers must be spread. This provides unbelievable results in all lymph disorders, including leukemia, lymphoma, and swelling in any part of the body. Hold for ten minutes, three to four times daily. The patient will soon feel a tingling left hand, then left foot, then right foot, then right arm, then heart. If the heart is not felt, hold a little longer after the right arm tingles. Some feel it as a warmth. The entire healing takes three minutes.

Venous System

To influence the entire venous system, hold the following points on the head. In the back of the head are two indentations just behind the ears. Hold them for three minutes at a time, two times or more daily. You will be amazed that the protruding veins in your hands will vanish.

Blood

The key position for the blood is as follows: The patient should lie on his/her back. You stand on the right side of the body. Lay your right hand over the liver, the left hand folding skin and muscles over the right hand. Start below and move slowly upward until you reach the stomach. Do this stroking and kneading 12 times, slowly and not harshly.

Lungs

The entrance key to the lung is on the right side, between the second and third rib. Hold this spot and take a deep breath. Exhale in a forceful manner. Do this seven times. It will stimulate the entire lung.

Exhaustion

The seat of exhaustion is situated four finger-widths below the navel. It is called Hara, an old Sanskrit word.

Place your left hand over Hara, right hand over left hand, and hold it that way. Breathe in slowly, bringing breath to forehead. Exhale forcefully, holding the tongue on the roof of the mouth. Do this breathing six times in a row.

Nervous System

The central nervous system has its keys below both knees. If your central nervous system is in trouble, as in back injuries or paralysis, start rubbing the places below your kneecaps. As soon as you can, get on your knees and start "walking" on your knees. In the beginning, it is very awkward and painful, but soon your central nervous system will respond. In some churches, kneeling benches are installed. These are very helpful to bring the central nervous system into action. In Europe, healing shrines are placed on high places, and there are no roads permitting access by car. People have to walk up. Better yet, they are instructed to crawl up on their knees. When they arrive, after hours of effort, they are healed.

Keys for Nervousness

First press the outside of both legs. Underneath the knee you will find an indentation, which is called the point of heavenly tranquility. Press this for five seconds. Next press on the middle of the back of the skull and count five seconds. Next press on the back of skull on both sides and count seven seconds. Next hold behind both sides of the jaw and count ten seconds. Cross your arms and hold points on back where scapula and humerus meet and count ten seconds. Do this twice daily.

Emotional Nervous System

The key position of your emotional nervous system is one inch below the breastbone. Hold this point until you feel a deep release, sometimes accompanied with a cracking sound.

Brain

Key position for the brain (three times daily): back of the skull, at the base, on both sides (hold for seven seconds); points on back (both shoulders) where scapula and humerus meet (hold for 30 seconds).

Ovaries

Key position for the ovaries: Heal your ovaries by holding your hands over the points on the inside of each leg, just below each knee. Very valuable in cases of tubular pregnancy. In that case, someone else should hold for 15 minutes. Apply black cohosh tincture.

Chapter Six

✳

GLANDS

"There is nothing hidden that shall not be revealed and nothing secret that shall not be known."

Our glands are important to overall health. They help regulate the complex functions of our bodies, maintain the chemical balance, secrete important hormones, and contribute to our mental and emotional well-being. The following information provides techniques for maintaining and improving the condition of our glands.

Pineal Gland

In the back of the head are two indentations just behind the ears. To stimulate the pineal gland, hold these points for 30 seconds two times daily.

WILD CHERRY BARK TINCTURE

This is food for the pineal gland; use seven drops twice daily.

Pituitary Gland

The pituitary gland is the master gland that controls the complex functions of the body. It is located in the middle of the head just below the brain. The output of the pituitary hormones control:

- Chemical balance
- Nerve impulses from the neighboring part of the brain called the hypothalamus
- Endocrine system and its secretions of hormones and enzymes

The tiny gland controls heartbeat, blood pressure, temperature, and the functions of the body that are not subject to conscious awareness. This pituitary gland with hypothalamus is the go-between for intellect/emotion and body functions.

To stimulate the pituitary gland, hold the forehead and the point one inch below the breastbone for 30 seconds.

Thymus Gland

The thymus gland is located behind the breastbone. This gland is next to the master gland, the most important gland in the body. The lower part of the thymus gland touches the upper part of the sac in which the heart pulsates, and the thymus influences the sensitivity of the heart. The thymus gland is the seat of the ethical and moral understanding of a person. When we become mean, this gland stops working, and doubt, fear, unethical behavior, and despair set in. The thymus contributes to inner faith, love, and strength, and it enriches our lives. Sodium fluoride causes the thymus to malfunction, and this adds to the destruction of the inner values such as faith, respect, free will, and hope.

The thymus gland has its ganglia at the back of the neck and from there extends to the brain along the fifth and sixth nerves, connecting eyes, ears, nose, and heart. The thymus gland excretes special hormones, from which all glands benefit. A child is born with a well-functioning thymus gland. It is happy, trusting, hopeful, and loving. The thymus and heart work together. But as a person gets older, if nothing is done to keep the thymus gland working, it barely makes the necessary hormones and secretions. The thymus gland shrinks, and rigidity sets in.

Rigid neck muscles	=	Shriveled up thymus
Rigid eyes	=	Cataracts
Rigid ears	=	Hearing problems

In the spiritual realm, this makes rigid dogma—lack of confidence in the goodness of our creator and a lack of confidence in ourselves. If the thymus functions normally, there is no such thing as a lack of courage, dissatisfaction, or faultfinding.

To strengthen this gland, beat the breastbone lightly with your fist and roll the head back and forth, up and down. Thyme tea is also highly recommended. Please stay away from waters and items containing sodium fluoride. Sodium fluoride has a direct controversial vibration for the health of the thymus gland.

WHAT TO DO

1. Pound it; massage it.
2. Vibrate it; rub it in a circular motion.

It will take up to nine months to revive the thymus gland.

Thyroid Gland

The thyroid regulates energy in cells, and it balances the cells as needed. The thyroid gives us material to strengthen our happiness, self-esteem, and hope. A slow-acting thyroid can be the cause of bones that will not heal. The face muscles sink in. Also, forgetfulness sets in. The interest in everyday doings diminishes. The voice becomes weak.

Low thyroid can contribute to:

- Hay fever
- Asthma
- Throat irritation
- Loss of voice

- Stomach trouble
- Constipation

THYROID STIMULATION METHOD

Have your patient sitting up for this application.

Right side application:
The healer stands on the right side, places the patient's left hand on the point at the middle of the clavicle, and the patient's right hand on the side of the neck just below the jaw. The healer does the same with his hands to supplement the energy. Hold these contacts for about one minute.

Left side application:
Get the patient to do the same thing on his left side, placing his right hand on the middle of the clavicle, and his left hand on the left side of the neck just below the jaw. The healer places his hands on patient's hands as well. Hold for one minute.

Spleen

The spleen is a very important organ. God planted it so deeply in our bodies so that nothing can happen to this delicate organ. It is the only organ in the body that has two auras. It is also the only organ to be in complete yin-yang balance.

I have studied every available book on the subject of the spleen. A blocked up, congested spleen is a mystery. It is a gland of inner secretion, and once the ducts become congested, we are in severe trouble.

An enlarged spleen (greatly the result of congestion) is capable of raising the left rib cage visibly. There is very little pain connected with it, but fullness and pressure. A sluggish, congested spleen can add to mental instability, depression, and stupor. A congested spleen makes a yellow complexion, and brown discoloration appears over eyes, cheeks, and around the mouth. It may affect the heartbeat, and often people sigh a lot.

Weakness; disorientation; and being afraid of people, cellars, darkness, or closed rooms point to troubles in the spleen. People with spleen trouble seem to be more affected by haunted houses and foreign energy possessions, and many are obsessed or possessed for years until a helping minister or a psychic steps in to release them.

To open the congested area of the spleen, the following method is extremely helpful:

Stand at the head of your worktable or slightly to the left of your friend. Place the fingertips of your right hand under the right armpit of your friend. Rest your left hand over his/her solar plexus. Hold your hands in this position until you feel heat or throbbing. Your left hand will feel it more distinctly. Watch the color coming into your friend's face. See the lines in the face smoothing out. Watch the dark discoloration go!

Do this seven days in a row. On the second day, the person may expel a sour, putrid stool, black or dark green in color.

Try this simple method on epileptics; those mentally confused or mentally exhausted; and on your friends with blood impurities, acne, wrinkles, or skin discolorations on the face and arms.

The spleen is the reservoir of stored electricity in the body. If the spleen is not in order, the brain takes over this job. However, this has one drawback—people become egocentric. They accomplish nothing worthwhile.

Note: Okra and red beets are revitalizing foods for the spleen.

Lymph Gland (Node)

The lymphatic system has many "pumps." If several of these pumps are stuck, they do not deliver the fluids to the special organs, and the organs become malnourished or toxic.

Cancer is now so widespread that Swedish massage therapy cannot be administered unless you know for sure a person has no cancer cells in the body. Otherwise, the cancer is spread from one place to another very, very quickly.

In order to influence the entire lymphatic system, the following treatment is needed.

Dr. Houston's Method

Spread the fingers of the left hand and rest them on the patient's neck. Make a spade with the right hand and go straight into the left armpit. Hold. Now relax and feel; imagine and direct with your prayers and your mind the proper flow of the lymphatic system. First, the left hand of your friend will become warm and cozy. Then the left foot, then the right foot, and then the right hand. You gave a complete massage without hurting in about three to five minutes.

When it comes to local lymphatic congestion, there are methods widely used. I demonstrate the most important ones. The lymph is a delicate matter. It should be handled gently, so lightly that you just touch the area in question and quiver your hand like a feather in the wind.

The entire lymphatic system is laced with filters—filters for the feet, tonsils, heart, arms, and brain.

See also chapter 5 (Key Positions: Lymphatic System).

Sacred American Indian Treatment

- Healer has both hands open over patient without touching.
- Patient has both hands open.
- Healer moves hands slowly up and down.
- Patient moves hands slowly up and down.
- Healer moves hands slowly sideways.
- Patient moves hands slowly sideways.
- Healer goes behind ears and sways hands back and forth.

The healer goes to the base of the skull and opens the lymphs. Then, the healer goes down the spine using both hands at the same time on the right and left, ever so slowly, one finger ahead of the others.

Tonsils

Hold one finger on the tip of the collarbone. With the other hand, "milk" the lymph gland down with a very light touch. Do it from the ears to the clavicles. After finishing this movement about 10 to 12 times, repeat on the other side.

Usually the sore throat is totally gone and the tonsils start shrinking. Do this as needed.

Breasts

Breast lumps can be removed at an early stage, without surgery, by stimulating the lymph flow. The woman stands, while a second person, preferably the male energy of her husband, does the following (for purposes of this example we will assume the lump is on the right side):

1. Stand on the right side of the standing patient. Put the spread fingers of the right hand on the right side of the sternum where the breast tissue attaches. Simultaneously put the spread fingers of the left hand on the right side of the spinal column, approximately parallel with the right hand. Hold for 90 seconds. Prayers for healing are entirely in order through these stages by both the subject and the practitioner.

2. While holding the left hand in the same place, move the right hand to a position directly in the armpit with the spread fingers extending straight down out of the armpit. Again hold for 60 seconds.

3. Return to the first position and hold for 60 seconds.

4. While holding the right hand in the same place on the right side of the sternum, shift the left hand to the position in the armpit and down from it. Hold for 60 seconds.

5. Return to the first position and hold for 60 seconds.

6. Repeat this process three times daily until three days after the lump disappears. If the lump is on the left side, substitute the words *right* and *left* in the above instructions. If the lump does not disappear in three weeks, the case is more advanced and needs different care, including the possible use of magnets or fungus-removing herbs. Of

course, there is always the possibility the lump is something other than a blockage of the lymph glands.

Adrenal Glands

The following exercise will stimulate the adrenal glands and encourage them to produce more natural cortisone.

Stand with your heels together. Inhale deeply and fully, then hold your breath. While holding your breath, turn your head to the right until your neck muscles are pulled as taut as possible. This must be done without moving the body. Stretch until you cannot turn any farther, then hold to the point of dizziness.

Now exhale through the mouth.

Repeat this process three times on the right side, then three times on the left side. Each time try to hold the taut muscles just a bit longer.

Pancreas

This large, elongated organ lies partially behind the stomach. It excretes three juices:

- A digestive juice that flows into the duodenum.
- Insulin for glucose digestion.
- Alcohol for nerve and brain function.

To keep this organ in good condition the following method would be helpful: Lie on your back. Start "aura" massaging from the left side down to the middle of the body. Do not touch the body. Keep hands one-half centimeter from the skin. Massage again and again for five to seven minutes, then bring your hands to the right side and stroke, not touching the body, 12 times up the middle. Give the person one-third teaspoon of ground nutmeg in 1 cup of hot water and let him sip slowly. The blockage hindering the flow of fluid to and from the organ will be lifted, and the organ will resume its work.

🝆 ❁ ⚶

Chapter Seven

❁

INNER ORGANS

"Life is given to us for the perfection of our nature and thus the betterment of mankind. The betterment of our nature cannot occur without honest labor."

To keep our organs in the best shape possible, we have to understand how they function and how they contribute to our general physical and emotional health.

The Kidneys

The druids considered the kidneys of animals sacred, and these were not eaten but buried under large oak trees. The bean-shaped organ must have impressed these people, or perhaps they had an inner knowledge about these valuable organs. In any case, these old-timers had respect for kidneys and their functions, and every year, they secured a large variety of herbs by drying and storing them for winter use. These herbs were shave grass and chamomile. Birch leaves and white nettle were dried, too, and in the fall, the druids gathered rosehips.

In the Middle Ages, shave grass was used widely, and in old writings, stories, and descriptions of herbs kept secretly in monasteries, shave grass was the number one remedy for kidney troubles. I found something very interesting about what these people did. They stuffed the mattresses of kidney sufferers with either male or female fern. I found a detailed description of when to use male fern and when to use female fern. Male fern was used when the right kidney was not functioning, female fern was used when the left kidney was not functioning. In later works on herbology of the Middle Ages (about 1806), distinguishing between female and male ferns was dropped, and people were just advised to sleep on ferns.

We all know that our kidneys are filters. When the kidney quits its job, we certainly are in for trouble. The waste and water is not carried away, and it builds up, fills the subcutaneous tissue, and eventually hinders the normal functioning of the human body. Dr. Alexis Carrel showed with the experiment of the chicken heart that, for life purposes, it is just as vital to feed the right nutrition as to carry away the waste material, and this is just what the kidney filters are designed for.

Going back to our old-timers, who distinguished between male and female remedies for the kidneys, I stumbled on a paper of a most modern scientist, a man whose knowledge and findings will be recognized 40 to 60 years from now. This man told me that the right kidney takes care of the waste below the middle of the body, which is yang in nature, and the left kidney takes care of the waste material of the upper part of the body. The difficulties in finding the proper remedies pertaining to kidney dysfunction seem to arise from our misunderstanding of their proper functioning.

We actually need two remedies—one for the malfunctioning of the right kidney and one for the malfunctioning of the left kidney. Here is where the knowledge of our old-timers comes into play. In some cases, they took female fern and related herbs and stuffed them in their bedsteads; in other cases, they used male fern. How they found out which kidney was at fault without our shining laboratories, our test tubes, our expensive outfits, is a riddle to me. In admiration, I search in these old books to compile new versions of old-time remedies, and with it I stumble over the most recent discoveries that will shake an old belief of kidney malfunctioning.

It is a fact that men suffer a great deal more from ailments of the right kidney and women more from ailments of the left kidney. It is peculiar that this is so and that no extra thought was ever given to the frequency of this phenomenon. While studying the works of a famous herbologist, I found that for restoring the functions of the right kidney, the following herbs are particularly beneficial: pumpkin seed tea, watermelon seed tea, shave grass tea, and male fern tea. For the left kidney, cornsilk, uva ursi, fresh watermelon, and female fern are more in order. When both kidneys are impaired in their functioning, chamomile tea should be taken and should continue to be taken a month after all signs of illness are gone.

The overworked kidney often expresses its dire need for attention in sore and painful knees. When it becomes painful to the knee to raise your foot from step to step on a stairway, see your physician and take a urine sample to him. Also, when your eyesight is dimmer in the mornings than in the evenings or when sparks appear at odd times of the day, take your urine to a laboratory to make sure your kidney is not involved.

How did people formerly find out when the kidneys were not functioning properly? They boiled one cup of the first morning's urine and added one teaspoon of vinegar. The urine would coagulate when albumin was present, and our old-timers took care of it with herbs. For albumin, they took motherwort. When the urine showed blood, they took shepherd's purse or marshmallow root. The latter was also used for burning urine.

The herb uva ursi is found in forests all over the world and is an old, old remedy for bladder trouble. It was used alone or in combinations with other herbs to relieve discomfort and promote healing of the urinary tract. The first time I saw it used was in the modern clinic of Professor Brauchle. He was so successful that many modern clinics adopted his suggestion, and it is widely used in gynecological sections of modern hospitals as a routine drink after operations or childbirth. With the help of this herbal tea, the time spent by nurses on catheter work was cut to one-fifth, and nurses, as well as patients, were relieved from this dreaded performance. I myself had to use the tea several times. It tastes bitter, but not undrinkable, and it should be taken hot. After the first eight ounces, a marked relief of tension is noticed and, taken every two hours, burning of the bladder soon leaves. Unfortunately, I could not interest any laboratory in finding out what it is that is of such great benefit. It could not be sheer suggestion. Gynecologists would not allow it in their clinics as a standard routine if it did not help to relieve discomfort, save time for nurses, and promote healing.

The Stomach

The stomach is an organ neither yin nor yang, neither positive nor negative, and has its own way of operating. There are 50,000 glands ready to dissolve, prepare, harmonize, liquefy, and electrify the food we take in. The stomach is very emotional. One notices this particularly in children. When they are upset, they complain of stomachache. Pain and discomfort somewhere else gives them pain in the stomach. Young women have a tendency to throw up, and men and women faint when seeing blood or emergencies, because the stomach contracts so suddenly that it shuts off all connections for a little while. Unfortunately, our stomachs are very abused nowadays, and the stomach's capacity for digesting the food we fill it with is greatly overtaxed. A cocktail stimulates the stomach glands, and these industrious little workers pour the acids, pepsin, hormones, and fluids into the stomach so that it is halfway filled before you sit down for dinner. And here comes a whole spectrum of mixtures—vegetables, fruit, pie, buns, steaks, ice cold water, potatoes, sour cream, butter, ice cream, and boiling hot coffee. We sink back into the chair and say, "That was good, I enjoyed the dinner. I am full and satisfied." Is your stomach satisfied, too? I doubt it. The muscles of the stomach will have to give so there is room to work—a worktable so to speak. But the gases of the mixture will start occupying the room, and the stomach muscles have to give some more. The ice water has paralyzed the production of pepsin. The hot coffee has numbed the nerve control. The mixtures start gassing, and the owner of the stomach has to have Alka Seltzer. Isn't that the way it goes?

When children come home from school after an active day, the first trip they make is to the refrigerator to fetch a glass of ice cold milk or ice cold juice. How wonderfully it quenches the thirst, how exciting it tastes. It rolls down so smooth and easy. Down there where it is dark, however, it is not so easy. The coldness contracts every one of the glands. The juices of the stomach, being acid in nature, are quickly neutralized by the alkalinity of the milk, and the cold cheese sits in those emotional children until very late. You wonder why Rose is so nervous, why Tim is so uneven in behavior, and why little Marge sits over her homework and cries. She is tired and emotionally wounded. She feels sick all over her whole little body. No wonder. The coldness in an overheated body gave a jerk to the whole nervous system. Some people are more robust than others and can take more of this punishment, but many break down early in life emotionally, and with a host of stomach disorders.

The stomach is made for simple, wholesome foods, not ice water and mixtures. Fruit and vegetables are incompatible at the same meal. In the East, they know the secrets of food combining and will not offer their families fruit and vegetables at the same meal. Fruits are air food, and vegetables are mineral food. Just keep them apart. Apples are neutral and can combine with either one or the other.

Wrong combinations and too much of all of it makes a thick, gluelike mucous in the stomach, and then the trouble begins. There is a wonderful recipe that I found in an old Swedish-Finnish herbal doctor book. It must be pretty old—printed in 1890, collected from folk medicine. Thirty minutes before a meal, take six ounces of warm water, add one tablespoon glycerin and one teaspoon ground hops. Hops happen to be full of natural pepsin. I converted this recipe. I bought liquid pepsin, and here is the modern version of this formula. Combine six ounces of warm water with one tablespoon of glycerin and one-half teaspoon pepsin; drink this thirty minutes before each meal. Taken long enough, it works and brings new life to the worn-out stomach.

As I said, the stomach is very emotional. Old folks and our best nutritionists all say do not eat when you are upset, angry, or full of hate. Your stomach is so emotional, it is crying for peace, understanding, and harmony. When you fill the stomach while you are full of hate, the stomach will not produce any digestive juices, and the food sits there and rots.

When you scold a child while he eats, immediately the stomach folds up its production of juices. Here you have the first onset of an ulcer. Love your child and his tender stomach nerves. The disciplinary words can be said much later. One of my dearest friends in New York had a very sensitive, beautiful, and intuitive boy. There were some minor marriage problems, however, and the parents were unable to come to an agreement about disciplinary procedures. One day the boy smashed a window. It was on a Friday. Bob wanted to confess it right away to his father, but the mother said, "Please do not do it now. Your father promised to take me out, and he will be so angry it will spoil my evening."

That evening Bob could not eat but was forced to empty his plate. That night he was almost sleepless. In the morning he dozed off, and he wet the bed. The father was already gone when Bob came to breakfast. Again he felt guilty—this time for wetting the bed. He could not eat, so he drank ice cold pop and waited for the evening to tell his father about the broken window, for which he knew he would get a severe spanking, which he did.

The child grew up. Many trips to the psychiatrist were made. Stomach ulcers developed early in life, and he now has to eat a carefully selected diet. Instead of a healthy, robust boy, he has become a timid hypochondriac.

Once stomach ulcers are established, your physician will tell you it comes from nerves, that pressure has built up, and now at last you listen and don't drink ice cold beverages any longer. Stomach ulcers can be deep and make little pain. The flat sores cause discomfort. The deep ones are more serious, of course. It is known that vitamin E heals without scars. The scars in a stomach are particularly unwanted because in the folds of the scars, new ulcers are ready to come up.

We all have the remedy for stomach ulcers in our kitchen—the lowly potato. Juice one potato with the same amount of warm water and drink before meals three times a day. You also can grate a potato on a grater and squeeze through a cloth. It just takes a little more time and a larger potato. Later on, a piece of raw potato chewed very thoroughly before a meal feels good and relaxing to anyone who has had stomach trouble or a weak stomach. The red potato is better for this purpose. Caution! Potato juice cannot stand at all. It has to be drunk right away. Of course, cabbage juice is so well known for its U factor but you need a juicer and organically grown cabbage. Otherwise, the result is doubtful.

The Liver

The liver is one of the organs greatly afflicted in this time and age, but there have been liver afflictions reported at all times. They used to call it biliousness, and when someone was listless, mentally disturbed, off his rocker, the old physicians said, "He is liverish."

The liver plays an important role in detoxifying the bloodstream and the lymphatic system. Besides this, the liver has many other functions. The function of detoxification is greatly overtaxed. When we breathe in the air, we also breathe in lead from car exhaust. With our food, we take in DDT, additives, and chemicals galore. Cooking in improper cookware, we add more insult to the liver. With sprayed vegetables, we add a dash of arsenic and other no-nos—small amounts, of course. What are we doing to counteract these poisons and help the liver? Not much. We continue our diet of fried foods, potato chips, cakes, pies, and cookies until one day the liver tells us, "I have had enough," and we start feeling sick. We were sick all the time, but now we feel it. As Dr. Donsbach said, "We used up all the power of the liver to detoxify and are approaching the last 20 percent of its capacity.

Liver trouble was known in all ages, but what did our forefathers do about it? There is a beautiful little story I read as a child that I have to relate. Once there was a very rich man whose only purpose in life seemed to be eating. He grew heavier and heavier and nastier and nastier. One day he became very ill and sent for the doctors. All the potions and pills did not help. He grew nastier, and the pain grew worse. Finally, he sent for a wise man in a faraway town. This man realized that no potion would do and sent him a letter telling him, "Friend, you have a big monster in your intestine. It will eat you up. Come and see me. You have to walk all the way and eat only hard-boiled eggs and greens." The frightened man started out. He was so heavy and tired. He walked only two miles that day, cursing and aching and crying. But every day he could walk more, and after weeks, when he reached his destination, he was slim and happy and whistling and full of vim and vigor. This is one way to cure biliousness.

LIVER AND GALLBLADDER EXERCISES

Hold the left hand on the right shoulder. Brush with the right hand 21 times from right side to the middle of the body (stomach).

Here's another exercise that's effective for maintaining a healthy liver. Slightly touching the skin, rub in half-moon fashion. Start at the side, just below the chest, and move your hand in toward the center. Work slowly, take your time. After you do this seven times, hold your right middle finger down on a spot just below the rib cage. Do this firmly. The congestion will break up, sometimes with a gurgling sound. Also, hold the person's right middle finger and at the same time hold just under clavicle (on the right).

The Lungs

We can remain without food for four to six weeks, without water for four to six days, and without air for four to six minutes. What is it that makes breathing so important? Why is it the least talked about subject? We all talk about good foods. Feasting and fasting are common subjects, and books are written about the tortures of being deprived of water. But few have described the agony of not getting enough air. We should be terribly concerned about breathing, but more so about the air we have to breathe.

The lung is a yin organ and is the opponent to the yang of the intestinal tract. Only because of this divinely intelligent arrangement of positive and negative, the body can live and have its being.

We all know how air is taken in through the nose and mouth into the lungs, how the gases interchange, and how we exhale, leaving the oxygen for future use in our bodies. Much less known, however, is the fact that, with every breath we take in, etheric energies are taken in, too. Now these etheric energies are what the yogi calls "prana," which is etheric. Prana is both positive and negative. It has two polarities, and our body is made to make use of these energies. Through the right nostril we inhale positive prana, through the left nostril we inhale negative prana. Both are needed for our well-being.

It is calculated that without the influence of prana, magnetic, and other forces, we could not live. We could eat day and night and starve to death on the seventh day because we could not extract enough energies from the food and drink we could take in. This is one explanation why some people can exist on very little food. Most often these are happy and balanced people, and they try forever to lose weight. They have an abundance of energies and are rosy cheeked and well-rounded. There are those who get so enveloped in the work they are doing (usually creative work) that they forget all about food and drink, yet they have all the energies they need to do the job. While they do their work, they forget the surroundings, but they do not forget to breathe, and it is a balanced breathing since they are happy and balanced. More etheric energy is, therefore, extracted from the air, and they experience no loss of weight or energy whatsoever.

When we inhale and fill our lungs with air, the etheric energy is extracted and drawn into the fourth-dimensional tubes that lie to the right and left side of the spine. The right tube is called *Pingala* and starts on the right nostril way up in the nose. *Ida* starts on the left nostril and extends down the left side of the spine. As I said, etheric energies are positive and negative, and Pingala draws the positive current, while Ida draws the negative current. We are made to draw these currents alternately. One hour we draw positive, and the next hour we draw negative. This is the way we are made, but when we let ourselves become disturbed emotionally, we bring this out of balance and neglect to draw the energies in the right proportions. The time we interchange from one current to the other is extremely important. These times are the creative moments of our day. In this flick of a moment, our thoughts are creative. It is in this moment that we experience the law of the astral universe—the law of the next dimension in which everything is formed by thought alone and in an instant.

This one flick of a moment in which we can manifest good or bad, love or hate, destruction or creation is so important that you should never find yourself having any bad thoughts or lingering on hate, destruction, death, fear, illness, or divorce. You might create it right there and then. "The fear will be upon you," said the Bible. Having only good thoughts at all times, to be ready for these moments of your day, should be your concern so that the energies will manifest in good and constructiveness, in selflessness and in advancement. We have to make ourselves ready for the Lord. All the churches teach that, and still they don't know that this moment comes to us every hour of our life.

We call the positive current of prana the solar energy, while the negative current is called the lunar energy. The solar energy being drawn through the right nostril is positive in nature and can be used for self-vitalization.

Place a piece of cotton in your left nostril and breathe only through the right nostril for about one hour. During that time use your thoughts. Center your thoughts upon the part of your body that needs rebuilding or rejuvenating. You will be surprised at what happens.

Mary T. had a very bad cold. All the aspirins could only soothe the headache that went with it. She felt miserable all over and called for help. Besides aspirin she had nothing in the house, no linden blossom tea, no lemons for fresh juice, not even vitamin C. Well, I told her to plug up her left nostril and to lie back to feel the healing take place. Sure enough, it took less than half an hour, and then Mary started to feel better, and she continued to do so. She returned to work the next day.

It is known that great natural healers breathe for greater periods through the right nostril than through the left nostril. They are able to use and extract more solar energy than other folks can and, therefore, cannot exhaust themselves readily.

We all know of people with a very low metabolism. Mr. Hildt hardly digested his food. Everything this poor man ate literally turned to poison. Gas discomfort, sour stomach, and miserable feelings after every meal, he hardly dared to sit down to the dinner table. Every day his wife turned the kitchen upside down to prepare, pulverize, grind, blend, peel, and juice his food. It did not get better. Mr. Hildt got weaker and weaker. One day he got a miserable cold. His left nostril was all blocked up, and he could only breathe through the right. This day his food digested well, and he felt fine in his stomach. He had plenty of time to think, and when the cold disappeared toward evening, he plugged up his left nostril and started to eat. Guess what? He experienced no discomfort. When he woke up next morning, he was hungry for the first time in a year, and his head felt better. By plugging up his left nostril, he balanced his polarities; the sluggish circulation stepped up, and he grew better and better.

We really should make a habit of breathing through the right nostril when we eat. The solar current, the positive prana, speeds up the process of metabolism, and we can digest and extract all the energy from the food we eat. We have to eat much less to be satisfied because we get so much more out of our food. On the other hand, in case you have to undergo a fast, plug up your right nostril and breathe more through the left. You will not be so hungry because it will slow down the metabolism in the body.

Ellen was always listless, anemic, run-down, constipated, and just not herself. She complained of lack of energy and dullness in her head. Treatments for anemia resulted only in temporary improvement. Everyone thought and said that she liked this condition. Her husband was a very fine person and realized that this was not the Ellen he knew. He asked for help, and I suggested she plug up her left nostril so more solar energy would enter her body. This was on a Friday. Sunday afternoon they took a long hike to the mountains and enjoyed every moment of it. She returned refreshed and with her lovely complexion all tinted pink from the new strength and new life force. She never needed another iron pill or B_{12} injection.

Now, we find individuals who have an excessively nervous temperament. Their metabolism is highly stepped up. Usually they are thin and restless and sometimes a little hard to get along with. These people would benefit greatly by breathing every day for an hour through the left nostril. The food would have time to be digested more slowly, and the stepped up metabolism would become more normalized.

On the other hand, we find people who have a tendency to breathe through the left nostril too much and may have a terrific water retention and weight problem. The left breath, the Ida center, is called the moon center. To a great degree it regulates the distribution of the various fluids and secretions of the endocrine glands and the water household of the body. Since the water in our system is highly polar in nature, it stands to reason that the lunar breath has an influence on the fluidic matter in the system. These people may try to breathe through the right nostril more often to balance weight and fluid matter more thoroughly.

When we think of the power of breath and how important it is in our life, it sounds strange that more importance is not placed on the study of taking in life currents, energies, and supplies for the body through the nostrils and the inexpensive way to attain the building stones for our bodies. Scientific breathing should be taught and practiced in every household. There is still a lot more to be accomplished with controlled breathing. Your demand for fresh, lead-free, unpolluted air is justified. In polluted, lead-laden, DDT-saturated air, the vital current of prana is reduced to 2 percent. Where are we supposed to get our energies from?

People with lung conditions are easily tired. Besides not enough oxygen, they cannot extract enough prana from the air. Why are there sanatoriums for lung diseases in Switzerland? If it were only oxygen that the incapacitated lung needed, all sanatoriums should be on the ocean. But at lower altitudes, lung patients cannot extract enough prana; therefore, they feel a lot better in the pure air of Switzerland. Theories are in circulation as to why Switzerland is so healing and uplifting, stimulating and different from other parts of the mountainous world. There is but one difference—the Alps have a lot more available prana than other mountains.

Lung Ailments

Coming to specific lung ailments, there are many treatments our forefathers used, and they were most successful in helping the sick. When lungs were congested, people grated onions and placed them between two layers of cloth. They applied this poultice to the front and the back of the chest and placed hot water bottles or heated stones over it.

Blessed thistle is one of the herbs used to reestablish the yin magnetic power of the lungs and is known to heal long-standing infections of the lungs.

Oatstraw, with its natural silicon, helps to strengthen the lungs. I heard of one mother who, after World War II when so many suffered from tuberculosis (TB), went out to gather the leftover stubbles in the oat fields. She boiled them and gave them to the children. None of her four children contracted TB in spite of all the contact they had with TB-infected neighbors.

The yin-yang harmony of lungs and intestine is interrupted, and all effort should be made to balance the disharmony. In America, we have the wonderful aloe vera plant, which the Indians used for shortness of breath. From the near East, fenugreek, the mucous solvent, is imported. Mullein leaves applied to the chest and brewed as a tea for drinking is a well-known treatment and is practiced in Europe and America. In old Greece, thyme, sarsaparilla, and marshmallow root were boiled in wine and sipped, and the chest was rubbed with hot pepper. All herbal teas that are good for the liver seem to be bitter. All herbs that are good for the lungs seem to be mild, and most of them are aromatic and very pleasant.

The tea of linden blossoms is an old-timer. In the Middle Ages, the linden tree was so appreciated that it was planted in almost every town square, and every little village had the center square planted with linden trees. There, the young folks met in the evenings for folk dancing and chats. In the daytime, young mothers met with the purpose of taking water out of the center well, and the old folks sat on the benches inhaling the fragrance of these blossoms.

Linden blossoms, taken right at the beginning of a chest cold, break up a cold after the second cup of tea. Care should be taken that you are well-covered because it induces sweat and breaks the congestion by opening the pores of the skin. Compresses of linden tea are healing in old wounds and eczema. The charcoal of the linden wood has something even more special. It neutralizes putrefaction in the colon and lungs, and it strengthens and heals. When there is no hope left for your patient, try the linden tree. Take one tablespoon of linden charcoal in powder form, place it in warm tea or soy milk, and drink this amount mornings and evenings for four to six weeks. The lungs will be so strengthened that all congestion will leave in a hurry.

The pine tree was used in the Middle Ages for relief of lung congestion. Branches of pines were placed under the bed of the sufferer. The young tops of pines were placed in a vessel covered with water and simmered for two hours. After removing the twigs, the juice was boiled for another hour to make it more concentrated by evaporation. Honey was added to preserve it, and it was boiled for another half hour. Placed in jars, it kept well for winter use.

Dr. Selig writes in his book *Krautergold* that the most healing are the branches of the creeping pine found high up in the mountains. Small branches are to be boiled for one hour. The brew is mixed into bathwater, and the patient takes a 15-minute bath. Rest is indicated after that. Sickly children and people with long-standing lung congestion are so strengthened that they become healthy after only a few weeks of this daily procedure.

I have seen miracles with pine concoctions concerning weakened lungs and weakened nervous systems. The sleep is deeper, breathing becomes regular and deeper after the first bath, and when you place twigs of pines under the bed and in the room, the volatile oil continues to heal 24 hours a day.

Whenever you see someone who cannot breathe easily, remember how lucky you are. Count your blessings. Forget the petty things that bother you, and ask angelic forces to help your suffering fellow man.

LUNG EXERCISES

The techniques of breathing are discussed in many yoga lessons. Some of them are so time-consuming that we Westerners with our quick actions lose patience. We do it once or twice and leave the rest to the yogi. Remember, however, when you inhale, you take in the pranic energies. Therefore, train yourself to inhale very slowly. You may exhale fast, but always inhale slowly. There are certain breaths that are used for the stimulation of the various functions of the body. We have mentioned some already. One to overcome mental lassitude and brain fatigue is very easy and can be done at any desk. Close both nostrils, inhale through the mouth, and then force the breath into the nasal passages and start to exhale with the mouth closed. When this is done, the etheric current is diverted and focused into the brain cells and acts to stimulate them. Do that several times in a row and several times a day.

Or you can try this exercise: Stand or sit with the spine erect. Place the tip of the tongue at the roof of the mouth or the root of the upper row of teeth. Then close both nostrils with the fingers and inhale slowly through the mouth. Take a long deep breath until you have filled the lungs with air to full capacity. The slower you inhale the more you can take. Then slowly exhale all the breath from your lungs through the mouth. Contract the abdomen at the same time. Do that ten times. This will increase the oxygen supply in your body.

Now relax. Pucker your lips just as you do when you are going to whistle. Then close the nostrils with the fingers. Slowly inhale a deep breath through the mouth. Close the mouth and exhale slowly through the nostrils. Draw through the mouth and exhale through the nostrils ten times. This is the second exercise for the oxygenation of the bloodstream, and it liberates the etheric current. The next one is very refreshing for the control of thought. Close the left nostril and inhale through the right. Count to eight while holding your breath. Preferably, take eight of your heartbeats as the amount of time. Exhale through the right nostril. Then close the right nostril and breathe through the left, count to eight while holding the breath and release through the left. Inhalation and exhalation is through the same nostril. This method will enable us to confront our problems and bring to definite and understandable conclusions that which was obscure, veiled, and in turmoil. Try it.

Another Tool of Harmony Is Breathing

When we breathe in, we are closer to God, to the universal presence. As we breathe in, we are receiving strength. As we breathe out, as we exhale, we are releasing old stuff that we do not need. As we breathe in, we should imagine a soft color such as pink, blue, or green. As we exhale, we should exhale used-up energies in darker colors. This will not only oxygenate our blood, but it will also spiritualize our being. Blood is the carrier of energies. Purified energies come in with the breath and uplift our mind and soul.

Note: Children and adults who walk with toes pointed inward are prone to lung diseases.

Circadian Rhythms Influence Organs

The biological clock that regulates day and night cycles is called the circadian rhythm. Besides color, the healing of congestion is rhythm. It is a tremendous healing factor. The heart heals under the rhythm of 3/4, the lungs under the rhythm of 2/4. The lymphatic system likes an even, soft rhythm like the sound and the rhythm of a brook in the forest.

Eat Light Food

- Rhythm of the heart: Every ½ hour give 4 oz. of distilled water for two days.

- Rhythm of the kidney: Every 15 minutes give a small piece of water-melon or pear for three days.

- Rhythm of stomach and colon: Every 50 minutes give 2 oz. of chlorophyll water for three days.

- Rhythm of the liver: Every 1½ hours give 10 oz. limeade for seven days.

- Rhythm of the pancreas: Every 45 minutes give ½ tsp. paprika in 2 oz. pineapple juice. Alternate with papaya juice. Do this for two days.

- Rhythm of the nerves: Every 60 minutes give thyme tea and 12 manukka raisins for one week.

- Rhythm of the lungs: Every 2 hours give 1 cup linden flower tea and chew 2 small pieces of calamus root on the hour when you do not drink tea. Use it like chewing gum. Spit it out after you chew it. Do this for three days.

Chapter Eight

❋

THE COCCYX

In my opinion, this chapter is the most important chapter of the entire book. A misaligned tailbone not only gives physical troubles, but it also adds heavily to psychological disorders. The coccyx is a pump that pumps fluids of the bone marrow, the spine, the brain, and other encased internal fluids that are necessary for health.

The Coccyx in Relation to the Inner Organs

The sacrum and coccyx connect anteriorly with the rectum—the prostate in men or the uterus in women (via Douglas's pouch)—and, further forward, with the bladder. These relationships are important in the treatment of many urogenital disorders.

The tailbone is surrounded by the anterior, posterior, and lateral sacrococcygeal ligaments. In the normal person, these ligaments allow good mobility while maintaining appropriate tension on the coccyx and associated structures. The coccygeal ligament is very important. It is the only manipulable ligament that enables one to have a direct effect on the dural tube.

Almost all the soft tissue of the pelvis is attached to the coccyx. These connections should make you aware of the sacrococcygeal articular lesion.

The waste of the lymphatic system and the waste gases of the nervous system leave the body via the tailbone. When the coccyx or tailbone is twisted, bent, or injured, these gases are held as in a cup. When released, suddenly these waste gases are thrown against the diaphragm, causing severe sudden illness, often mistaken for a heart attack.

Why does the coccyx have such wide-ranging effects? Because it is a pump. Suppose, for example, at 2 or 3 A.M., you experience severe pain in the heart region. You are rushed to the hospital just to be told that it was a pseudo heart attack. You are told that you are anxious, upset, and overworked.

What happened? The malfunctioning coccyx could not take care of the overwhelming nerve poisons in the system, and the heart was sent into spasms.

Fears, frustrations, phobias, and depression tend to create excessive alkalinity over a period of time. The cerebrospinal fluid and the sympathetic chasm join together by the vagus nerve. The trigger point is the coccyx, the tailbone. If the tailbone is out of balance, these emotions can take over and make life most uncomfortable for the sufferer.

Psychological Disorders

- In depression, always check the sacrum and coccyx.
- In brain fog or loss of clarity, see if the tailbone is in place.
- Check for poison in the tailbone.
- Check for parasites lodged in the tailbone.
- In leukemia, check the tailbone.

Poison in the Tailbone

- Lead deposits lodged in the tailbone prevent the coccyx—the pump—from full action. Lead deposits can cause epilepsy and other nerve disorders.

- Mercury iodide lodged in the tailbone is one of the causes of shaking.

- Nickel lodged in the tailbone can be the cause of pain over the entire body. Sit on a small pillow filled with poppy seeds.

- Parasites lodged in the tailbone can cause insanity and lunatic behavior. Mix equal parts oil of wintergreen with oil of sassafras.

Apply a few drops of this mixture to the tailbone. It will take several weeks to see results.

In all cases of leukemia, the tailbone should be checked and realigned. This information comes from Dr. Brauchle; he began using these nonmedical methods in Dresden, Germany. In one wing of a 2,000-bed hospital, he worked with 25 patients a week, mostly children. Each week, 25 patients would walk out perfectly healed. Not one died from leukemia.

Then and now, both science and medicine dismissed his results. They called these methods hocus-pocus magic, witchcraft, or some kind of hypnotherapy. It is none of these. We call it the healing power of God. Over 5,000 people who had leukemia used these methods and continued living. They call it *wonderful*.

During World War II, this amazing hospital was destroyed along with the healing practice. Only three people who had this knowledge escaped. I was one of those people, and I eventually moved to the United States, where I keep the methods alive on a modest scale.

The realignment of the coccyx is not painful; you cannot make mistakes. It is not an osteopathic or chiropractic treatment. It stands all by itself as a vibrational treatment. When the tailbone is realigned, it gives a whooping spurt of energy to children.

How can coccygeal problems happen?

It may have happened with a fall on the coccyx bone many years ago, in a car accident, by giving birth, or other circumstances. This is what osteopathy is teaching us, and they add in their books: This coccyx trouble has its effect on the kidney, bladder, lungs, stomach, heart, and other organs. We do not understand this completely and more research has to be done.

Remember the coccyx is a pump for bone marrow and all other liquids encased in the tissue of bones.

How can you align a tailbone?

Put the patient on his or her stomach and loosen the spine by light massage downward on both sides of the spine. Do this three times on each side.

Turn the patient's head so it is facing you. Hold one hand over the sacrum. Lift the leg farthest from you, bend the knee and bring it toward you (inside), and then back to the middle. Do this three times. Bring it three times outside and back to the middle, then three times down and back to middle, and then three times up and back to the middle.

Now turn the patient's head the other way. Repeat: three times inside, three times outside, three times down, and three times up.

Then, lift the leg by sliding a hand under the thigh, and swing the leg toward you three times. Repeat all the steps on the other leg.

Chapter Nine

❋

THE SPINE

To accomplish anything, we have to have faith in ourselves. Very few people have faith in themselves. They like to put faith in other people, and then they are shattered when other people do not live up to their expectations. Have faith in the power of God that lives in you. When we want to accomplish something, we have to have a definite goal. Remember, a true goal is a channel of service.

Disk Trouble

Use St. John's wort oil remedy for disk deterioration. Have the person lie on his or her stomach. Have two people stretch the back. The person at the upper back stretches the muscles up toward the head while the second person stretches the lower back muscles down toward the tailbone. Then, rub St. John's wort oil on the spine; otherwise the adjustment will not hold.

Adjusting Ribs

Three people work together on this one—the patient and two helpers.

The person with the rib out sits on a chair and relaxes. The first helper counts "1-2-3-UP!" On the word UP, the patient should blow out his breath. Not too deep a breath, just regular breathing. Do this four times.

While standing at the patient's left side, the second helper holds the patient's arm at his side, elbow bent. The helper's left hand is under the patient's left forearm, and his right hand is under the patient's elbow. When the first helper counts "1-2-3-UP!" the second helper lifts up on the patient's left arm. Do not pull the arm away from the body. Push up from the forearm and elbow points, raising the entire arm and shoulder three to five inches or so.

The first helper, while standing on the (now-standing) patient's right side, places four fingers of the right hand on top of the rib cage near the center of the body on the patient's chest. Then, he places four fingers of the left hand on the top of the rib cage near the spine on the patient's back. As the helper counts "1-2-3-UP!" he uses a rotating motion by pushing with his right hand and pulling with his left hand to put the rib in place. This rotating motion may need to be done in the opposite direction as well, pushing with the left hand and pulling with the right hand, but not very often. The helper then moves down the rib cage to a lower spot and repeats this motion three more times, each time going a little lower on the rib cage. The helpers should switch sides and adjust the other side of the patient's body in the same manner.

Bringing the Clavicle into Balance

When the muscles on the inside of the arms are hurting, always remember the collarbone is out! If you do not have a chiropractor, someone has to help you. Sit straight on a chair. Interlace your fingers, bring your arms to shoulder height, and place your thumbs on the clavicles. Your helper can do the job now. From behind, the helper slips his left arm underneath your left arm and holds your wrist. Now the helper swings you backward three times. Have the other side done three times also. If arm muscles are still painful, repeat. Measure the clavicles, and you will find that they are straight.

Hips

The hips are so important because they are the foundation that the entire spine rests on. If the hips are not in place, spinal adjustments will not hold for very long. Also, when the muscles that hold the spine in place have arsenic poisoning or cadmium poisoning, then the poison will bring the spine out of balance.

First determine the position of the pelvis. This is done on each side by placing the hand, palm downward, on the crest of the ilium. This lets you know which is the low side and which is the high side. You are ready to correct this.

Step 1—Stand with your feet spread comfortably apart. Place your hand on the low side on top of your head. Bend forward and rotate in a 45-degree arc. Move sideways and up on the side, with your hand on top of your head. Shake the hips back and forth.

Step 2—Without moving the feet and keeping them apart, lift the toes of the high side and rotate on the heel inward to pigeon-toe the foot. Now place the hand on the high side on top of your head. Bend at the waist, forward, down, around, and up, inscribing a 45-degree arc. Retrace this 45-degree arc back to center. Shake hips again.

Step 3—Place both feet together and do the low side once more. Then, retrace this 45-degree arc back to center. Drop both hands to the sides. Shake shoulders back and forth. Measure your hips and you will find that they are okay.

Whiplash

European method: Press the patient's body from the side with 50 pounds of pressure. Lift the patient just off the floor quickly. Then, go to other side and do the same. Whiplash is gone.

Aligning Knees and Ankles

With one hand, hold the patient's ankle. Bend and hold the knee with your other hand. Lift the patient's leg to the middle and bend it inward with moderate pressure and tension. First rotate it inside, then outside, and then straight down. Do this three to four times.

Putting the Spine in Place

The patient sits on a chair, with both hands on top of the head. He moves 45 degrees forward, then to the right side, and up. Then, he moves 45 degrees forward, to the left side, and up. While the patient moves, the helper slides the vertebrae into place.

Mastoids

The mastoids have much to do with our hearing. The two mastoid bones are connected by tissue. This tissue extends forward making a connection with the inner eardrum. The outer eardrums, right and left, make connections with the mastoid glands, which are directly behind them. These glands are not as noticeable in children as they are in older people. If there is an interference in the ears caused by the mastoid glands, it also interferes with our sight, taste, and smell. If the skull is deformed or out of order, it will bring pressure to bear on the mastoid glands, interfering with the medulla, and also affecting the senses of taste and smell. The seat of sight is located in the back of the head near the mastoid bones. If there is an unnatural pressure on this bone, it will dim the eyesight.

In many cases of eruption in the mastoid bones, a fever or inflammation may appear. This causes a soreness of the bone behind the ear, an enlargement of the mastoid glands, and, finally, interferes with the tongue and throat. One gland from each mastoid extends down the throat and attaches to the collarbone. A feverish condition of the mastoids may result in many disorders and throat trouble, causing large deposits of phlegm or mucous in the throat. You may recognize these conditions by a very bad odor in the nostrils.

This will be well appreciated by all patients who are unfortunate enough to suffer with sinus and migraine headache symptoms, loss of sight, or loss of hearing.

To remedy this, the patient should lie down on his stomach on a table, with the helper standing on the patient's left, and the patient facing right. The helper holds the patient's left thumb between his right thumb and fingers and places the fingers of his left hand on the right side of patient's head, just below the ear.

The process is then repeated on the other side. The patient turns his head to the left, and the helper stands on the right side. The helper takes the patient's right thumb between the fingers and thumb of his left hand and places his right fingers on the left side of patient's head, just below the ear.

Carpal Tunnel Syndrome

To help this syndrome, massage from the small finger upward. Move stroke by stroke up toward the thumb. Do this ten times. Hold the point on the inside of the wrist just above the thumb and rotate wrist. The tensed ligament goes in place.

Chapter Ten

※

MUSCLES AND TENDONS

U se the following methods for maintaining fitness in your muscles and tendons. Energy and flexibility are important aspects of a healthy mind and body. Understanding contact points and how to apply pressure with fingertips and hands allows us to heal ourselves and others.

Muscle Tone in Arms and Legs

Follow this method to assist the muscle tone in both arms and legs:

The person should lie on his back. The helper stands on the person's right side. The helper then places the fingertips of the right hand on the patient's right palm. He also places the fingertips and thumb of the left hand on the point halfway between the underarm and the neck.

Energizing Muscles

LOWER LIMB ENERGIZING

To energize lower limbs, place the palm of your left hand over the back of the patient's left knee and your right hand over the back of the right knee. If you want to give yourself a treatment, the same procedure can be done while seated, using your own palms to make the contacts behind your own knees.

AMERICAN INDIAN METHOD

Here are some methods the American Indians used. Stand on the left side of the person you want to give energies to. Take the middle finger of your right hand and place it under the skull on the right side of your patron.

The left hand you place on the area you want to give energies to—a broken foot, a stomachache, or wherever energies are needed. Hold it there for five minutes or until the pain is relieved.

In order to increase the power, do the following. Stand on the left side of the person you want to give energies to. Place your middle finger of the right hand under the skull as before. Rest the left hand on the solar plexus. Another person places his left hand over yours and his right hand over the hurting or injured body part. This method is excellent. The joining of powers triples and quadruples the healing action of the laying on of hands.

Leg Cramps

These contact treatments will greatly assist in all cases of leg cramping that usually occur due to a calcium deficiency. The patient should lie down on his back. The healer stands on the right side of the patient and places the fingers of his right hand on the patient's right side on the outside edge where the hip and leg meet, and he places the fingers of his left hand on the right shoulder of patient. The same procedure is carried out with the healer on patient's left side. Each point is held for about 30 seconds.

Abdominal Energy Release

The use of the following contacts will release tension in the regions of the stomach, colon, and small intestines.

The patient should lie on his back. The healer stands on the patient's left side. He places the fingertips of his right hand on the left side about two inches above the navel. He then places his left fingertips behind patient's left knee.

The patient can use his hands to do the same to boost the energies—the left hand is held behind the knee—but the right hand moves one inch higher from the navel to make contact, and then one inch lower than the first contact on left side of the navel.

The same procedure is carried out with the healer standing on the patient's right side. The healer uses the fingertips of his left hand for abdominal contact on the patient's right side and places his right fingertips behind the patient's knee.

The abdomen will feel relaxed and thus help the energy from the abdominal brain (the navel) to become effective.

Hip Tension Release

Using these contacts will assist in producing a marked relaxation of tension in the back of the neck muscles. Patient should lie on his stomach and face right. The healer stands on the patient's right side and places his right hand fingers and thumb on the patient's right palm, and then on the neck just under the right ear. The patient can reinforce the energy of the healer, or he can give himself the contact treatment.

Chapter Eleven

Magnetism

Science teaches us that different bodies can occupy the same space if these bodies are on different vibrational levels. For example, our surrounding atmosphere is filled with light waves, sound waves, heat waves, odic force, electricity, magnetism, gases, water vapor, and many unsolved mysteries. But none of these collide, explode, or interfere with each other, because they operate on different vibrational levels and rates. You know that many calls can be made through one telephone line at the same time because each call is sent on a different vibrational rate.

The same is true in the human body. As far as we know now, we have five bodies. They occupy the same space but vibrate on different levels. There is the physical body. It is the body we see and feel, the body that hurts when we pinch it, the body whose bones can break and whose skin can be injured by pressure or knife. The medical physician is well trained to take care of this body.

Another body is the mental body. It cannot be seen, felt, cut with a knife, bent, broken, beaten up, or stamped on, but it occupies the same space as the physical body and psychiatrists are trained to help when this mental body needs help.

Churches preoccupy themselves with the understanding and teaching of the spiritual body, and chiropractors are trained to take care of the coarse electromotive body of the human machine. The coarse electromotive body runs through the nervous system and has its stem in the spinal column. By keeping this spinal column and other nerve paths in good health, the chiropractor helps his patients achieve good electromotivation of the finer body; therefore, better circulation of the physical body.

There is one more force occupying the same space as our physical body. This has no name as yet, so we call it "Gauss magnetics." It is of finer electromotive vibration, and it has its seat in the lymphatic system of our body. There, in the lymphatics, it can be contacted by pressure or with the Chinese method of acupuncture. This finest of the five bodies, as we know it now, bridges the gap between the physical, as our allopathic doctors know, and the spiritual, as the churches teach and know about. It is the body that carries universal electric force through our system, and we all know that without these universal high vibrational forces, there would be no life possible.

The Gauss magnetics is a body that contacts every cell and every nerve in our body. It is the true blueprint after which life form takes place. Through the finest, intangible channels, the power of the universe has its being. The universal force enters through the left hand, passes by will through the right hand and involuntarily through the right foot back to the earth and universe. That means we can direct the universal force by will through our right hand to heal and soothe and balance conditions that are out of order. If we do not exercise will, the force flows through us and leaves the body through the right foot.

Up to now the existence of Gauss magnetics was denied because no channel has ever been found on a cadaver. Postmortems do not show any such channels. The reason for this is that the lymphatic system and the channels collapse at once at death. However, there are 20 chains known, and any stoppage in one of these chains may result in physical or mental difficulties. Gauss magnetics has been known to the Chinese people for centuries. They call it acupuncture. Acupuncture, as the Chinese teach and use it, is designed to open blocked channels in this finest of our bodies. There is no doubt that with intense studies, feeling, and intuition, these people have developed a healing system par excellence that works for the Eastern races. Unfortunately, the puncturing of the skin with different needles, gold, silver and others, to different depths of the tissue does not have the same desired quick-healing result in people of the Western hemisphere. I often wondered why and asked and observed until one Japanese physician told me that the Westerners have a slightly different physiological makeup, and the finer bodies cannot be reached by acupuncture in the same satisfactory way as in the Easterner. That means we have to get busy and find our own way to contact the channels of Gauss magnetics.

The Bible talks about contact healing in several passages, and I often wondered what this is all about. I felt that there was a deep understanding and a deeper meaning in these passages, and it had to do with the "laying on of hands." However, when the laying on of hands is done in a scientific manner by knowing the passages of Gauss magnetics, by contacting important points of this system, the laying on of hands becomes an art of grace and knowledge. Every physician can use the old-time method of the Bible to the greatest benefit of his clientele.

I am eternally grateful to God for bringing me in contact with an American physician who, through divine guidance, found the keyboard to Gauss magnetics (contact healing) for us Westerners. His name is Rev. Dr. Fred M. Houston, who developed a scientific method to open the finest of our bodies through contact by hand and fingertip. When the channels of Gauss magnetics are blocked, stopped up, reversed or otherwise not functioning, contact healing comes to the rescue. It is the Western way of acupuncture. As acupuncture brings reliable results to Chinese and Japanese people when Gauss magnetics is involved, contact healing brings reliable results to us Westerners when Gauss magnetics needs help.

Magnetism, as used in healing, had been known throughout the dark ages, and before that, every civilization gap went back to the use of magnetism for healing. By magnetism, I do not mean hypnosis. These are two entirely different subjects. Hypnosis is the use of mind matter for one particular task. For example, there is self-hypnosis. You tell yourself one word or sentence or idea over and over until you believe it, and it becomes a part of yourself. Or someone else hypnotizes you. He puts his mind force over your mind force like a darkening cloud, and you cannot establish your own pattern of thought. Like all forces, it can be used for good or bad, constructively or destructively, or for healing or destroying.

Magnetism is, scientifically speaking, the mitro-genetic power, the mitro-genetic rays of the human body. These rays are found to be created between the frontal lobes of the brain. When the frontal lobes are closer together, more of the mitro-genetic rays are released. Quantity and quality depend and change with the polarities of the body. Magnetism is not electricity, even so it acts similarly. It is, as one schools states, an offshoot of electricity released by the body.

In the East, the magnetic energy is called the Astral Fire. If one has a sufficient amount of Astral Fire, he is vital, alive with attractive personality, and he attracts things to him because magnetic quantity will attract greater quantities.

Now pause and, in your thoughts, go to visit your partners, your friends, and yourself. Here is the secretary—vivacious, happy, of utmost efficiency, kind, and considerate. Her activity is contagious, her smile genuine, her work is done like a breeze in sunshine. Next in your acquaintances is the listless man—always tired, neurotic, nagging, never happy, without glow and shine. Another of your friends is the old couple—always ready to help and comfort; early mornings they take a walk or tend the garden, and neighbors pause to chat and receive their magnetism and grace with a bunch of flowers or a basket of fruit. And here is Nelly—the woman who only talks of her illnesses and failures along the road; she sees the thistles in her garden but not the flowers, and strangely enough, all sorts of mishaps are following her path of life.

Coming back to the manifestation of this magnetic energy in our body, we understand that the mitro-genetic rays are formed between the two frontal lobes of the brain. The quantity can even be measured. Some people have a great deal more magnetic power released than others. This is the reason that some have more natural healing power than others. Everyone has healing power. Every mother can soothe her child in pain, fear, or agony. Every loving hand can release headaches, tenseness, and disharmony.

Science neglected magnetism and concentrated solely on electricity. Magnetism, however, has immensely greater possibilities for mankind, particularly in healing the sick. Some of us have trained ourselves in long hours of work to direct and release the healing emanation through the right hand and, therefore, to have more results than others. However, the healing power is in all of us.

There is another power joining the mitro-genetic waves generated between the frontal lobes of the brain. This is the earth magnetism. This power and strength is free for the taking and can be used at will. It enters through the left hand, is magnified and made usable in the seat of the mitro-genetic wave and can be directed by will. It emanates through the right eye, the right hand, the right hip and the right foot.

At Cornell University, a discovery was made that emanation, either from the right hand or right eye, might destroy the microorganisms of yeast. They found that when those emanations are directed by the will, the time required to destroy the microorganisms is considerably reduced.

Magnetic healing is not spiritual healing. Magnetism is a power that science knows to exist. It has not been made workable as electricity, which has been put to many uses. Science found out that magnetic energy is of a certain definite octave of vibration. For instance, human magnetism, the mitro-genetic waves, vibrates within the infrared rays and is detectable with instruments that are adjustable to the reception of this particular wavelength.

Magnetic force influences the psychometer (pendulum) and is based on the magnetic stream of the universe. In the fine optic instruments used to photograph the planets, magnetic energy is put to use. Water dowsing and other arts have been practiced for centuries. We have just forgotten how to use the magnetic forces in this day and age.

In case of blood clotting, one well known physician uses only magnetic healing. He sits on the left side of the patient, whose legs are flexed. Never touching the body, he places his right hand over the head. His left hand is two inches away from the tailbone.

I myself have witnessed blood clots disappearing, disintegrating in less than 20 minutes. My sister was dying. A two-inch blood clot had lodged one inch in front of her heart. The clouds of death already shadowed her face and consciousness. Her family was standing around, crying and in horror when I applied magnetic healing in the above described manner. To enforce our strength, we lined up one behind the other, lightly touching each other. After several minutes of silence we all heard something burst. My sister let out a scream. The blood clot had traveled through the heart in small pieces and she lived.

In South America, the old Incas held the seeds they wanted to plant in their left hand and blessed them with the right. They installed magnetic powers into the seeds to influence the future crop. We bless with the right hand because we release the mitro-genetic waves with the right hand and install the spoken word of love.

Before we go into the practical application of magnetism, I have to say one word about the polarities of the body. The quantity and quality of magnetic power depend upon and change with the polarities of the body. The right side of the body is positive, the left side of the body is negative. This does not mean good or bad by any means, these are only polarities. Nothing in the universe exists without the polarities of positive and negative. The faculties of the two sides of the body are:

Right Side	Left Side
male	female
square	round and curved
blue	gold
positive	negative
physical	spiritual
cold	warm
hard	soft
aggressive	loving
perpendicular	creative

Magnetic energy also is the carrier of vibration. It is the energy that carries the thought to the various parts of the body and is the carrier of thought into our affairs. The magnetic energy in a healthy person can be seen as a very faint, grayish blue radiance. Light a pair of candles and hold a black cloth in back of your hands. Place the fingertips together and slowly pull them apart. You can see little wavy streaks coming out from the fingertips against the background. This is the color of the vibration of the magnetic energy.

The magnetic energy that is in our body has the power of healing. Of course, it is not the only power there is, but many people can be returned to the road to health with the use of the magnetic healing rays.

If we build a pattern of sickness in our mind, this pattern passes into the magnetic stream and is carried to different parts of the body, forming congestions that we could not get otherwise. Therefore, in all schools of esoteric teaching, much stress is laid on correct thinking. The magnetic force is the carrier of thought to the different parts of the body. The cells and the glandular system are influenced by thinking through the magnetic force.

My friend's daughter, Barbara, 17 years old, began to fail in health. Severe headaches and vomiting spells increased from day to day in frequency and her vision was blurred. "Possible brain tumor" was the physician's findings and hospitalization was scheduled. Next evening my friend called me to ask if I could stay with Barbara a few hours since she was at the end of her rope. I gladly went and found a restless, emaciated girl pounding her head against the pillow in agony. I sent my friend to bed and pulled a chair close. By placing my left hand over the girl's forehead, I picked up the congestion and let it run out through my right hand, which I lowered to the floor. With all my mind and heart I concentrated on the flow of magnetic force through my hands. In my left hand I felt a tremendous heat building up. I felt a force pulling my right hand lower and jerking it at times. I felt a tremendous uplift, as if the room was full of holiness and divine beings.

The girl calmed down. The tortured features smoothed out slowly. In a low voice, I recited the Lord's Prayer, and under the impact of this tremendous vibration, she closed her eyes and deep, regular breathing showed that finally she found some rest. I held my hand in the described manner for one hour and twenty minutes. Then I reversed it. I placed my right hand over her forehead, and with the left palm up, I gathered the magnetic stream of the universe and directed it with prayer to her aching head. A steady stream of strength ran through both of us. A warmth of indescribable nature warmed and uplifted us, and the greatness of God's wonder filled the house. Next morning the headache was much better, and after several days, Barbara could go back to her tasks.

Since that time, I tried it on myself. When a fruit can fell on my foot, I picked up the pain with my left hand to let it run out to the right. A burn was treated the same way. A delivery man mashed his finger in my door. It was ugly looking—blue, swollen, and painful. I held his injured finger in my left hand and let the magnetic flow run down my lowered right one. The pain left, the swelling went down, and he continued working.

The Western world has, as yet, only touched the surface of knowledge regarding human magnetism. Five thousand years ago in India, a book was written by Charaka called *Aynna Veda System*. In it is not only the perfect knowledge of material function of the body, but also the magnetic functioning of the body. So this is not new.

The practical use of magnetic energies, as explained, has been used as long as mankind has existed. However, in the Middle Ages, this knowledge came into discredit and was connected with evil, the devil, the dark forces. The churches burned many men and women who dared to heal wounds and sicknesses in animals and men through magnetism. Knowledge of hygiene was not in existence at that time, and these poor people died by the thousands or healed themselves in secret places with herbs and magnetism.

Science now recognizes the unseen powers of the universe, and the mysteries of magnetism can be revealed and made workable in our lives.

Mr. Wulf was in class. He was always cold. His hands felt like ice. In a warm room he wore two sweaters. Our teacher reached over and placed an eye cap over his right eye. "Just tell us what you feel," he said. Five minutes passed when Mr. Wulf took off one of his sweaters, saying nothing. In another five minutes he said, "My feet are as warm as toast. I never had them this way." We all rushed over to feel his hands and his feet. Sure enough the polarities had changed and equalized in his body to an extent that normal temperature was obvious.

In the same class was a lady sitting isolated, close to the window, which she opened off and on to release the heat, as she said. An eye patch on her left eye made her cool down in less than five minutes. She joined the crowd and was comfortable after that. In both cases the polarities had been in imbalance. One was overfunctioning on the right side, the cold side, the refrigerator side. The woman was out of balance with polarity on her left side. The simple application of an eye patch brought, in both cases, normalcy.

There is a simple way of increasing energy. This is very good if you are tired. Raise hands overhead. Close your right hand, keep the left one open and raise on your toes taking a deep breath. Let down and exhale; do this three times. You can also increase your energy any minute in your day by holding the left hand out to gather the magnetic force of the universe and, with the right hand held over your head, return it to yourself like a blessing from above. Be patient and do not touch your head. You might not feel the energy building up in your left hand the very first time.

There are herbs known to have more Astral Fire than others. The plant mistletoe, for example. The ancient druids considered mistletoe a holy plant, and they used it for healing and many other things. They found it to contain a great amount of Astral Fire. Also, the Canadian thistle and gotu kola, the herb from India, have more Astral Fire than any other plant.

In our exhausting modes of life, all of us complain of loss of energy, loss of vitality. Speed pills, coffee, tea, cigarettes, Coca-Cola, sugar and alcohol are consumed in enormous quantities. Why? Because we all feel a lack of energy; we are exhausted and run down. Could it be that, in our city life, we lost the connection to the source of magnetism? Our forefathers walked over a live green meadow. We tramp dead asphalt. Our grandmothers tended the garden and picked live roses. We dust artificial roses in our vases. Our grandparents ate live whole grains; we eat plastic, artificial, devitalized foods. We've lost our connection to the ever-renewing forces of the magnetic flow.

Part II

DIETARY NEEDS AND FASTS

Chapter Twelve

HEALTHY FOODS/HEALTHY BODY

Healthy food is not plastic, refined, puffed up, stabilized, or chemicalized for appearance, preservation, or shelf life. It is not overcooked or undercooked. Healthy food is not bleached and sprayed as in cereals and grains; it is not green picked fruits, meat with diethylstilbestrol, eggs from chickens fed with speed and hormones, nor milk in cartons treated with formaldehyde.

Healthy food is just plain, good food. With this plain, good food, the intestinal tract is able to manufacture its own vitamins (with the exception of vitamin C):

> B-vitamins
> Folic acid
> Pantothenic acid
> Biotin
> Methionine
> Rutin
> Vitamin K_2
> Vitamin P
> Niacin
> Converts carotene to vitamin A

However, the sterilization of the intestinal tract through preservatives, antibiotics, and unhealthy food hinders the flora from manufacturing these vitamins in sufficient amounts or, in some cases, completely.

Sincere efforts should be made to establish the balance of flora in the intestines by avoiding preservatives and by taking the following:

> Buttermilk
> Yogurt
> Sprouted foods
> Acidophilus cultures
> Acidophilus capsules

It will take several weeks and often months to reestablish the balance.

Until the intestinal flora is functioning to full capacity, all nutrients, which ordinarily are manufactured in the intestinal tract, have to be taken into the body by means of food supplements; otherwise, one, two, or multiple deficiencies will arise.

Food Combinations

Simple food combinations are a must to make the stomach work properly. With every meal you can change your menu. You can prepare 3 × 365 dishes and menus a year. Serve only three or four things at a time, but change with every meal and you will have a healthy family. I call it the "Trinity Diet." For example:

Breakfast: cereal, cream, and sweet fruit
         or egg or toast and tea
         or meat, vegetable, and tea
         or vegetable soup and bread
Lunch: salad and fish
         or meat and one cooked vegetable
         or potato and vegetable
         or fruit pie and carob drink
         or high protein drink and fruit
Supper: the same simplicity of one vegetable, one protein, and one salad;
         or potato, vegetable, and salad

Remember:

1) Never eat meat and milk at the same meal.
2) Never eat fruit and vegetables at the same meal.
3) Never eat acid fruit and cereal at the same meal.

Meat and milk need two different digestive enzymes. Since Moses' time, no Hebrew serves milk and meat together, and these smart people keep this rule very strictly. Fruit is cleansing, and vegetable is building. Fruit is yin, vegetable is yang. When both are put together, you have a mess. It is incompatible with your electromagnetic field. Acid fruit and cereal make a gluelike mixture and stick to the stomach lining, and children suffer from it. Give fruit or a healthful sweet between meals (after about two hours), and your little folks will be ready for a simple meal two hours later. Fruit juice and milk are food and have to undergo digestion. When children are thirsty, give them water.

I first was struck with food combining while working in the mission field. We had arranged a picnic to which we invited about 300 villagers. We celebrated Dr. Clark's birthday, and it was his desire to invite the villagers. We had salad, hot dishes, cakes, cookies, and hot and cold drinks. The people filled their plates with three to four items and let their children have no more than three items on the plate. When I filled my plate with all the goodies I saw, one woman shook her head and said, "How is your stomach going to react? You will bring tears to your mother's eyes." Being seventeen, I ignored this warning. By nineteen, I had a good-sized ulcer and terrible emotional upsets. I was raised on Spartan principles, and I negotiated myself into illness by trying to be smarter than my parents and disregarded the simple rules of health that I saw practiced right before my eyes. Only Spartan simplicity in the choice of food brought me back to health.

In Europe, there are special resorts for healing stomach ulcers, and this is their diet:

For the first days, eat nothing but carrots, cooked and mashed.

On the fourth day:
Morning:	carrot soup
Mid-morning:	potato broth
Noon:	potato and carrot

Mid-afternoon:	herbal tea, cream, and rice crackers
Evening:	carrots and baked potato
Bedtime:	herbal tea and cream

After one week on this regimen, most people can increase their food intake to a normal, productive diet.

Food Energies

Eat for energy! Refer to the following list to determine positive, negative, and neutral foods and food combinations. Always beat/stir your food clockwise.

Apples: Are neutral and go with everything. Good to "eat an apple a day."

Apple skin: It has osmium, which is food for the brain. Make apple skin tea for kids before they go to school, and the kids will learn better. Affects the brain and nervous system.

Bread and
  Vegetables: Good combination.

Coffee: It is neutral. When milk is added, it becomes negative. Same with white sugar. If honey is added, it becomes positive. If you're tired in the morning, take a cup of coffee with honey to open up all the glands. No more than one cup a day.

Eggshell: Easily assimilated calcium. Put eggshells in apple cider vinegar and drink after they dissolve.

Fruit and
  Vegetables: No energy.

Grains: Too much can cause allergies.

Meat and
  Bread: No energy when combined. It will take at least two hours
                  for energy to return. Cheese and/or eggs with bread the
                  same.

Meat and
  Potato: Good combination.

Oats: Keeps the immune system going.

Peas: Separate from other vegetables, especially carrots.

Rice: Universal, neutral food, but it is not protein.

Tomato: Take out the core of the tomato, since the core is nega-
                  tive. The tomato is positive. Eat two to three times a
                  week.

Naturally Occurring Disease-Fighting Substances in Food

Apricots	Carotenoids
Basil	Monoterpenes
Beets	Anticarcinogenic hormone
Berries	Catechins, Flavonoids, Phenolic acids
Broccoli	Monoterpenes, Phenolic acid, Plant sterols
Brussels sprouts	Indoles
Cabbage	Flavonoids, Indoles, Phenolic acids, Plant sterols
Cantaloupe	Carotenoids
Carrots	Carotenoids, Coumarins, Flavonoids, Monoterpenes, Phenolic acids, Phthalides, Polyacetylenes
Celery	Phthalides, Polyacetylenes
Citrus Fruits	Carotenoids, Coumarins, Flavonoids, Monoterpenes, Phenolic acid, Triterpenoids
Cucumbers	Flavonoids, Monoterpenes, Plant sterols
Eggplant	Flavonoids, Monoterpenes, Phenolic acids, Plant sterols
Flaxseed	Alpha-linolenic acid
Grains (whole)	Phenolic acids, Plant sterols

Grapefruit (red)	Lycopene
Green tea	Catechins
Horseradish	Isothiniocyanates
Kale	Carotenoids, Indoles
Licorice root extract	Triterpenoids
Mint	Monoterpenes
Mustard	Isothiniocyanates
Parsley	Carotenoids, Coumarins, Flavonoids, Monoterpenes, Phenolic acids, Phthalides, Polyacetylenes
Peppers	Flavonoids, Monoterpenes, Phenolic acids, Plant sterols
Radish	Isothiniocyanates
Soy products	Alpha-linolenic acid, Flavonoids, Plant sterols, Triterpenoids
Spinach	Carotenoids
Squash	Flavonoids, Monoterpenes, Plant sterols
Sweet potatoes	Carotenoids
Tomatoes	Flavonoids, Lycopene, Monoterpenes, Phenolic acid, Plant sterols
Turnip greens	Carotenoids
Walnuts	Alpha-linolenic acid
Winter squash	Carotenoids
Yams	Carotenoids, Flavonoids, Monoterpenes, Plant sterols

Chapter Thirteen

FATIGUE AND LECITHIN

There is physically nothing wrong with you. Your heart beats its steady pace; your lungs are able to inhale deeply. Your blood is in good order. Kidneys are functioning, and yet, you push yourself with every step. Every task becomes a nightmare, and just plain thinking is an effort that you would rather put off until tomorrow. You are fatigued, exhausted, depressed, and bitter and helpless against the nightmare of this experience. We have all had it at one time or another—after giving birth to a baby, after an operation, or after a long, long sorrow. It is like a shadow monster that comes over you. You want to escape by sleeping, but you wake up tired. You want to lick it by eating; however, after every meal you feel worse. You go to a movie, a dance, but you have to return early for want of rest. Pep pills make the situation worse in the long run, and sleeping pills you don't need. You become a burden to your surroundings and friends, and in their eyes, you can see what they think. "Gosh, she is just pretending; there is nothing wrong with her."

We find the descriptions of fatigue in many old-time medical books. I own one that was published in 1806, and it tells the same story, but they called it nerve fever, remarking that no fever is present. Strange name isn't it? We are more simplified and call it fatigue or exhaustion. The astounding part of this fatigue business is that even very young folks seem to suffer from fatigue. The effort to study or work seems too hard for them, and their brain-fogged condition is due to fatigue.

Let's put some light on this problem. We are out of energy when our adrenal glands decide to provide us with less cortisone or when we have mal-treated this perfectly good organ with too many no-no foods. Now there are very simple ways to give more specific food to this organ so that enough cortisone can be manufactured. The lowly alfalfa seed was used for centuries to battle fatigue. Soak three tablespoons of alfalfa seed in one quart water overnight. Next morning bring to a boil and simmer for ten minutes. Drink as a breakfast drink with a little salt. Drink the rest without salt during the day. Blend two tablespoons sunflower seed and ten dates in one cup of water. This restores energy beautifully. Pantothenic acid and vitamin C are foods for the adrenal glands. Damiana leaves are a great help to restore nerve energies, but one of the most important factors is lecithin.

What is lecithin? As far back as 1846, a chemist, M. Gabley, isolated a fat-soluble substance from egg yolk that he called lecithin. Forty years later, Y. L. Thudichum found a similar substance in brain tissue that he called cephalin. Fifty years later, these findings were reevaluated by two chemists, Schneider and Faleh. These chemists brought lecithin to the attention of the world. Lecithin is a compound of over 70 components. It belongs to the group of phosphatides because of its glycerin-bound phosphorus.

Lecithin is found in plant life, such as seeds and yeast, and is particular-ly abundant in soybeans. It is found in animals. Blood cells, spinal cord, and brain tissue are especially rich in lecithin. Organically raised eggs also have an abundance of lecithin. The human brain contains 28 percent lecithin, and the spinal cord has not less than 25 percent. Every nerve is surrounded by a sheath that also contains 25 percent lecithin. Lecithin is abundant in heart tis-sue, and the liver cannot function without it. Every cell wall has lecithin, and a network of lecithin is inside every cell wall. Here it is found in connection with protein; therefore, lecithin in this coalition is called lipoprotein.

Lecithin influences the structure of the protoplasm. It regulates the permeability of the cell walls. It is needed in carbohydrate, fat, and protein digestion, and it is a balancing factor in the acid-alkalinity measure of the body. Lecithin, as mentioned, is needed for the metabolism of the nerve. That means no nerve vitality without lecithin. No wonder we are fatigued. The body is not equipped to handle as much extra strain as our present mode of life prescribes. Unless we supply our chemistry with extra lecithin, extra choline, and extra unsaturated fats, we cannot have the extra nerve pep we need.

A healthy body is able to make the different components for lecithin in the digestive tract and liver. However, to bind these components together to form lecithin, we have to induce linoleic acid and choline. These two are the synergists, the spark that ties everything together to the compound called lecithin. That means that we have to have cold-pressed oils and extra choline in our diets.

When should extra lecithin be taken and in what form? There is a crude oil on the market, cheap and terrible tasting and full of lecithin and linoleic acid. However, this lecithin is fat-bound and not desirable for the emulsifying process of cholesterol. It is already fat-bound and will not do you the favor of loosening its liaison to combine with the highly fat-saturated cholesterol. The linoleic acid, however, will (if your intake of choline is sufficient) help you form your own lecithin. Therefore, it is a preventive measure and should be evaluated only as such.

Lecithin in dry form was found accidentally during World War II when every ounce of fat had to be extracted for human consumption. This residue, as they thought it was, took on new dimensions in the industry. First, the chocolate industry got hold of it and found that this substance took care of the fat problem in their product without altering the taste. It emulsified the fats, so you were not aware that there was fat in chocolate, and that made the product easier to digest. The candy industry was next, and so the demand grew and grew. Now lecithin is one of the weapons against high cholesterol, acting by emulsifying the fat in the body, veins, and arteries, by supplying an easily digestible, easily absorbent choline. By introducing cephalin to the heart muscle, it helps prevent heart fatigue. The brain tissue is especially grateful for more cephalin in the diet. It also increases the peristaltic action of the intestines.

In 1952, Dr. Stefan found that injuries to the brain were greatly helped by lecithin. Patients with concussions and traumatic brain weaknesses improved in weeks instead of months when lecithin was given. It was given in a dry form.

We should assume that lecithin, as it is, either in oil or granules, would be readily absorbed and used by the nervous system. It is so obvious when nerve exhaustion needs lecithin that lecithin should be given. However, both lecithin in crude oil form and lecithin in dry form have to undergo the enzymatic action of the digestive tract and cannot reach the necessary nerves in these forms. You know you need lecithin; your nerves are on edge; you are exhausted, fatigued, and beaten down, but the nerves cannot be reached by your simply eating lecithin granules or swallowing oil.

The enlightening work of Antom and Swanson shed light on this problem and gave us help through their fabulous discoveries. They found that lecithin can be absorbed directly into the bloodstream if a lecithin molecule is smaller than a micron. Then they found a manufacturer who reduced the lecithin to a microdifferential, dispersible form, and guess what! The exhaustion problem was licked. The nerve food was found. Lecithin in this form does not have to undergo digestive enzymatic action, but is carried right to the bloodstream and, from there, to the sheaths surrounding the nerves, brain, and spinal cord.

We do not need case histories on this subject. All of us are exhausted at times without reason. Sleep does not restore vitality; a cup of coffee seems to pick you up, only to let you sink deeper in fatigue afterwards. Why not try the new, exciting lecithin therapy? Our grandmother gave us egg yolks with honey, but she made sure that the yolks were dark orange. The light-colored egg yolks were not used. I remember her buying calf brain for one of the members of the family, and it was lightly steamed and served with orange-colored raw egg yolks. I guess her common sense told her to feed lecithin for exhaustion, and she saw results. However, our mode of living has increased the need for lecithin tremendously, and the orange-colored egg yolks are not available any longer. So, thanks to the tremendous discoveries and the manufacturers, we can get our lecithin nerve food on the market. Lecithin is found in the following:

Lecithin in oil—prevention.
Lecithin in granules—fat-emulsifying.
Lecithin in microdifferential form—the new, exciting nerve food.
Lecithin available as a combination of lecithin and whey; or powdered
        lecithin.

Lecithin is an important part of our diet. It will steady our nervous system, carry us over times of exhaustion, and make every day of our lives worth experiencing.

Chapter Fourteen

About Fasting

About 2,500 years ago, Hippocrates, the Father of Medicine, lived in Greece. His wisdom, knowledge, and experience were so outstanding that medicine today still honors him. Hippocrates founded the humoral medicine and therapy, which teaches that illness is caused by the humors being out of balance. If you wish to improve the health of the body, everything should be done to improve the health of the humors—to bring them into balance.

Much later, from 1821 to 1902, came Virchow with his cellular medicine. The greatness and newness of his discovery overshadowed the wisdom of Hippocrates. However, Hippocrates' followers were always active even when they were laughed at and persecuted. The theory and experience that sickness and illness cannot manifest in a healthy body and in a healthy blood and lymph system has brought great scientists and great physicians to use their heads and work out plans for us laymen so that we may be able to prevent illness. Prevention is the goal, and preventive medicine was originated by Hippocrates.

The human body consists of more than nine-tenths fluid. Some of the fluid is bound in the cells and is a substance of the cells. Some of the fluid, such as lymph fluid, blood fluid, and juices of the hormone cycle, are outside of the cells and bathe the cells, so to speak, from the outside. According to the different tasks of the humors (which means fluids), they have different appearances and different colors: light red, dark red, transparent, milky, and so forth. Because of the fluid and moving state of these different humors, it stands to reason that they interchange and exchange with each other and that they also permeate every cell and every organ of the living body.

There is no doubt that different organs finally break down when a continuous stream of unhealthy, undernourished, and impoverished fluids surrounds and penetrates them. "Nutrients being preserved with chemicals will stay preserved to a large percentage in the body," Professor Brauchle warned.

Nutrition overloaded with sweets will weaken the humoral fluid greatly. Nutrients lacking in minerals will neither restore nor prevent anything. The loss of minerals in some fluids, such as urine, saliva, and perspiration, has to be made up daily.

We have four to five quarts of blood and about two quarts of lymph fluid. In 24 hours, we produce one and one half quarts of saliva, two and one half quarts of stomach juices, one quart of gall, and three quarts of intestinal juices. All of these fluids end up in the intestinal tract. From there, they are reabsorbed and purified for reuse. Only about two to three quarts leave the body daily, and this has to be replaced daily. If we continually replace these missing fluids with soda water, Coca-Cola, sugar syrups, and other nonnutritional liquids, we soon will reap what we have sewn.

What is fasting? Fasting is a willful abstinence from solid foods, and sometimes liquids, and it is done for a specific purpose. Fasting has been practiced since mankind began. Many passages in the Bible show that in Biblical times people used fasts. These people used it mainly for spiritual reasons. They prepared themselves to walk with the Lord by conquering their carnal desires and practiced it in periodic fasting.

Many religions have maintained strict rules over the centuries about food intake and occasional fasting. For example, the followers of Islam never touch pork—maybe because of the danger of possible trichinosis. They are also forbidden to drink alcoholic beverages. The Catholic church still observes the Lent season, and its followers abstain from meat and sweets for several weeks. As time passed, people found that fasting was important not only for religious reasons, but for increasing will power by deliberately, willfully staying away from solid foods. Many powerful national, religious, and social leaders make a point of abstaining from food for several days at a time, just to clarify their thinking, to increase their will power, and to become better people.

Fasting is not synonymous with starvation. Starvation is a slow, painful process of dying while the body consumes itself. "With starvation you become a meat eater by eating, digesting, and consuming your own body," Dr. Carlton Federicks stated.

I had the privilege and the great fortune to have known Professor Brauchle, a man of great foresight and love, who directed a 1,200-bed hospital in Dresden. Most of the patients were treated by natural methods: baths, fasting, diets, therapeutic massage, herbs, and vitamins. Some of them were treated, in addition to natural methods, with allopathic procedures. The most happy combinations, however, occurred when Professor Brauchle started to employ men and women to sit down with patients and discuss their inner problems. These workers strengthened the will power of the patient, helped them to overcome doubts and difficulties, hate-filled and destructive thoughts, and reestablished hope and peace.

In his interesting and famous lectures, Professor Brauchle taught us that fasting is equal to a surgeon's knife. It does away with accumulated toxins of all kinds. In his lectures, he told of case history after case history where, under scientific, supervised fasting, people returned to perfect health. He continued to say that a raw food diet is the weapon of a physician for internal medicine and that a mixed diet is for the working man.

Now, if fasting is a physician's knife, we have to ask ourselves what it is that we want to correct. A surgeon does not perform an appendectomy when he wants to take out tonsils. He uses different methods to achieve different ends. A fast, therefore, must be in line with our intentions. Just to say "I am staying away from food" is neither purposeful nor scientific. Therefore, when you want to undergo a fast, ask yourself, "What do I want to achieve? Do I want to get rid of a certain affliction? Do I want to walk closer with God? Do I want to lose weight? What do I want?"

Mankind has invented many fasts. The Turks fast on delicious watermelons once a year; the Bulgarians on yogurt. The Romans drank mineral spring water. These old-time fasts are not scientific and are undertaken more or less because of tradition—just as grandmother gave sulfur and molasses every spring to every member of the family. Whether needed or not, everyone got a spoonful of molasses twice a day for a week or more. We have to become scientific and specific when it comes to fasting. It must be purposeful and meaningful. It must help our bodies—not destroy our bodies. It must support the efforts of an attending physician. It should be done only for a short period of time and with the full acceptance of the inner self. To that end, I have included several time-proven, purposeful, scientific fasts that are mainly used in Europe and administered in the clinics of famous physicians.

A fast on water alone, as it was advocated and practiced 30 years ago, was safe and effective at that time. Not so today. In our fatty tissue, all of us have accumulated DDT and other matter. A water fast loosens these foreign accumulations, but instead of pushing them through the liver into the intestine, they are driven into the bone marrow. This is the last place you want poisons to accumulate.

Dr. Buchinger, a man who prescribed fasts to thousands of people with great success, uses fresh pressed juices. This means freshly pressed fruits or vegetables. The juice must be diluted with water, half and half, or you may drink one glass of juice and one glass water at the same time. This is greatly used in cases of infectious disease, hypertension, leg ulcers, kidney disorders, skin diseases, and rheumatic diseases.

When you fast on your own, never do it longer than four days at a time and only once or twice a month if needed. Never use fruit and vegetable juices at the same time. You may alternate them. Always take one or two enemas a day if undertaking a juice fast.

One requisite is to take it easy during a fast. If you can afford it, stay only half days on your job or take the first part of your vacation for this purpose. Secondly, don't feel sorry for yourself. Your food will taste better afterwards, and you will feel so good just because you conquered the carnal man in you. Before you start a fast, consign your mind to it. Don't you make up your mind before you undergo an operation? Surely you do, and you know some parts of it are not so pleasant. Just feel yourself being wheeled into the operating room; the very thought of it gives everyone the chills. Some parts of fasting are not so pleasant either, particularly the first three days when the poisons loosen from the subcutaneous tissue. But again, the first three days after an operation are not so pleasant either. In any case, make up your mind and don't allow an uncle, aunt, neighbor, or anyone else to change your opinion. Perhaps it is best not to discuss it, just do it!

Rice Diet for Waterlogged Condition

Take one cup brown rice (short grain is preferred because it has more minerals). Wash it and put it in two cups of boiling water without salt. Boil for

35 minutes on low heat. This kind of rice is to be eaten whenever one is hungry. At noon and night, some applesauce or stewed pears without sugar might be added. Or you may boil some wheat germ and middlings in water and use as you would the above recipe. For best results, do it for five to seven days.

How and why does this diet work? When the sodium, which is in the fluid surrounding a cell, is out of balance with the potassium, which is supposed to be in the cell, fluid builds up. The fluid is kept in proper proportion and harmony through the positive and negative electricity of the two opponents and components, sodium and potassium. When the sodium decides to pay a visit to the potassium in the cell, the potassium will leave. The sodium, which has no business in the cell, cannot handle the incoming fluid, and you become waterlogged.

Fasting for Spiritual Reasons

Fasting for spiritual reasons is practiced widely in our society. It is, however, a fad in which people tend to fast senselessly for prolonged periods of time. They go on water fasts, the worst thing they can do, and overdraw their fasting capacity to the point of delayed return or even no return. Do not go on water fasts. The shortcut to fasting for spiritual reasons is the following, approved method. It is very, very effective.

Take one pound of manukka raisins and soak them in four quarts of water (distilled preferred) for 24 hours. Stir frequently and drink one to one and one-half quarts of the water in small sips in the morning from 7 A.M. to 11 A.M or 8 A.M to noon. For one hour take neither food nor drink and have lunch consisting of vegetables and salad with fish, eggs, or cheese. The supper is your choice of food but should not be taken later than 6 P.M. Do this for two to four weeks, or as you feel it is necessary. Meditate for short periods, five to ten minutes, several times a day. It is not the length, it is the depth that counts for us Westerners.

You may also use 36 ounces of grape juice in the above described manner; however, you have to add six ounces of water to the 36 ounces of grape juice in order for it to work. Why? I don't know. It must be a secret of the electromagnetic field about which we know little.

Three-Day Fast for Nerves

It takes will power and authority to stay on a diet, especially when your nerves give out. Practicing the following routine for only three days in a row will make a better "boss," a stronger personality out of you. After that, one day a week or one day every two weeks will keep your nerves sweet.

In one pint of cottage cheese mix three tablespoons almond oil or safflower oil and two egg yolks. Mix well and either make it sweet with honey or spicy with onions, salt, and herbs. Also, boil four tablespoons of barley in two quarts of water for 35 minutes. Strain and add honey and lime or lemon juice to the barley water so it tastes good.

Before breakfast: one cup of warm barley water
Breakfast: prepared cottage cheese; carrots, raw or cooked
Mid-morning: barley water
Noon: steamed zucchini; cooked green beans; cottage cheese, spicy
Mid-afternoon: barley water
Evening: cottage cheese; zucchini, stewed or baked; dish of barley, carrot salad; barley water
Bedtime: barley water, calcium tablets

Fasting for Kidney Ailments

Boil crushed watermelon seeds, one cup to three quarts water, for three minutes. Strain and store two quarts in the refrigerator while leaving the rest on the table. Every hour, take one-third cup of this lukewarm tea. For breakfast take watermelon. For lunch take acidophilous milk and/or yogurt, vegetable and raw food, some fish or egg, and rye bread. Supper is stewed pears or applesauce with yogurt or soy milk, as much as you like. Do this diet for three days, but continue watermelon seed tea and watermelon breakfasts for 14 days.

This recipe comes from Turkey. It was given to my mother by a prominent religious authority. I have given away this recipe many times. Every time the result was immediate and astounding. It balances the fluids in the system by releasing electrical currents and reestablishing the yin-yang function of the kidneys.

Super Diet

Using clay for healing is as old as mankind. Even the Bible tells us how Jesus took clay for healing the sick and as a medium of his divine power.

The mud baths used in European health spas are famous. These special clays, or muds, are full of natural hormones and vitamins E, A, and B-complex. There are thankful women who, after taking a series of baths, return to health and youth, singing praises to mud treatments.

In Europe, Luvas Healing Earth "Heilerde" is sold in drugstores. Every household has it in the medicine cabinet. For upset stomachs, people take one-half teaspoon in one glass of water. For diarrhea, they take one teaspoon in one-half glass of water. For food poisoning, they take it every half hour. For sore feet, they put it in the foot bathwater. For skin eruptions, they make a thin paste and apply that. In our hospital in Dresden, we used it on old sores. We just powdered them with clay dust.

Volcanic ash is a cheap and versatile home remedy. It was first used on a great scale by the British army. During the Balkan War, mortality from cholera was terrific. Sixty percent of all soldiers who contracted this disease died. When solutions of volcanic ash were introduced, the mortality rate went down to 3 percent. Since then, the British army has used clay for the treatment of acute food poisoning.

How does volcanic ash work? According to leading experts on geology, volcanic ash has one of the world's smallest molecules. These molecules are shaped like calling cards. The two broad surfaces have a negative electrical attraction, while the edges are positive. Therefore, volcanic ash can pick up many times its own weight of positively charged ions. Certain toxins and bacteria found at times in the body, and in the alimentary tract in particular, are of positive charge. Volcanic ash absorbs or neutralizes such intruders, and in this way, volcanic ash aids in the detoxification of the alimentary canal. It took an ingenious American man to realize these facts and to have the foresight to bring a product on the market that everyone can use with confidence and to full benefit. He took volcanic ash and emulsified it in a truly ingenious way. His product stays in suspension and does not settle to the bottom of the bottle.

The experiments of Dr. Howard E. Lind on the subject of hydrated water-suspended bentonite (volcanic ash) are extremely fascinating. They bring into scientific terms what our forefathers knew by experience. In his laboratory, Dr. Lind experimented with volcanic ash. He placed a 4,095,000-bacteria count in a medium and covered it with hydrated bentonite. After 60 minutes, the count was reduced to 2,495,000. After 90 minutes there were only 620,000 left. He made many other experiments with equal success and found that volcanic ash even neutralizes the dreaded staph bacillus.

Whenever the problem of health is partially or totally due to a toxic, overloaded alimentary tract, the following scientific and very effective fast should be considered.

Take two to three tablespoons of liquid bentonite in one glass of water.
Take one heaping teaspoon of detox or psyllium seed or intestinal
     cleanser (a bulk-making item) in one glass of unsweetened juice.
Drink more fluids, such as herb tea or water, afterward so that you
     have a total fluid intake of 16 ounces.

Do this five times a day: 7 A.M., 10 A.M., 1 P.M., 4 P.M., and 7 P.M. At 9 P.M., take an enema to eliminate all the waste from your colon so you may sleep soundly. On the fourth or fifth day, you will lose, besides long ropes of waste, black matter, which is the sign that you may start adding food to your diet such as some raw and steamed vegetables and raw and steamed fruit. Discontinue clay after the seventh day, reestablish friendly bacteria with acidophilus or yogurt and go on a good, natural diet.

This fast is modern. It is without hunger pangs. It is effective and help-ful, and it cooperates beautifully with your physician's suggestions. In case you need an operation, it is much easier for a surgeon to work when the ali-mentary tract is free of old waste. I know by experience as a nurse how unhap-py surgeons are when an overloaded "wastebasket" alimentary tract hinders and holds up proper surgical procedures.

Some time ago, I talked to an undertaker to find out what his side of the big tragedy was and what he had to contribute to help mankind. His biggest concern was the putrefaction of the alimentary canal. He said there are people with sixty pounds of waste in their intestine. They choked to death, he said.

That did it. The next morning I went on the clay diet. I was not hungry at all and worked all day long feeling happier and happier. On the third day the stool looked like long ropes of old waste, rubberlike and terrible. The old pockets had been emptying. Stuff sitting there for years and glued to the intestinal walls loosened out. Most probably the white gluten bread I used for two years had baked to the intestinal walls. Since that time, twice a year I go on a three-day clay diet just to have my intestinal tract in the best shape possible.

Mrs. R. told me her story and experience on this matter. She was 54 years old when it started. She complained of pain in her legs. Since she was somewhat on the heavy side, all tests were made for diabetes and similar ailments. She stopped smoking, lived on diet products for losing weight, and got worse and worse. A year later her right leg was blue and discolored and both legs were swollen and painful—no circulation. After six more months of intense suffering, amputation of the right leg was suggested. Someone had told her about the healing clay, and Mrs. R. started the very same day. For seven days, the old waste, accumulated from years of constipation, poured out. With every day she felt stronger. On her seventh day, the pain in her legs was gone. There was still some swelling and discoloration, she said, but she could walk. So she walked to the dress shop and shoe store to buy herself a new outfit for a new lease on life.

Cleansing Diet for the Liver, Pancreas, and Upper Intestinal Tract

Use the following regimen for cleansing the inner organs:

On first arising: one-half grapefruit (if hungry)
Breakfast: all the cooked or canned whole tomatoes you wish
Mid-morning: one whole grapefruit
Noon meal: same as breakfast
Mid-afternoon: one whole grapefruit
Dinner meal: same as noon meal
Bedtime: one-half grapefruit (if hungry)

Eat nothing but the above for four to seven days, depending on the conditions or poison. This is very good and should not disturb the patient. In some cases this diet will bring on a fever as the body starts to throw off the poison. This is also good and should not disturb the patient.

World-famous Dr. Evers, whose diet reform brings many multiple sclerosis patients back to health and walking, does this almost with diet alone. He teaches his patients how to sprout wheat and rye. His patients can eat these sprouts twice a day. He gives them hazelnuts, walnuts, sunflower seed, coconut, Brazil nuts, raw eggs, and raw milk. For fresh fruits, he gives them apples, pears, plums, cherries, and all berries. For sweets, the patients can have raisins, dates, and figs. For vegetables, Dr. Evers gives only those that grow underground, such as carrots, radishes, red beets, etc. For starches he gives whole wheat, rye bread, and raw rolled oats. With this diet, which is full of life enzyme, a drastic change in the sluggish metabolism is achieved, and Dr. Evers has results.

FOR LIVER ONLY

First day, on arising, drink eight ounces of hot water with fresh lemons squeezed into it. From then on drink the juice for breakfast, lunch, dinner, and whenever hungry. Also, stewed tomatoes and tomato juice may be taken, because it is also a cleanser. Drink hot water and lemon or tomato juice whenever you feel like it, the more the better. Do not worry about the following day because it is the same procedure.

It is amazing how hungry you become, so at bedtime on the second day, you will look forward to the following cocktail:

3 oz. olive oil
2 oz. castor oil
3 oz. whip cream

Be ready for sleep and be relaxed. Drink before bed and you may chew a little piece of lemon afterwards, just for taste. It is a lot easier than it sounds! At 3 or 4 A.M., you will answer nature's call, and in all your life, you will not have experienced so much dark and ugly smelling waste.

The next morning have the following breakfast:

Stewed tomatoes: Take ripe tomatoes and cut out the place where the stem is because this part of the plant is not fit to eat and, in most cases, is poisonous. (Tomatoes belong to the berry family, and you can core out the stem from strawberries, too.) Cut tomatoes in little pieces, add a little water and simmer them slowly. You may add salt, onions, or seasoning, but no fat of any kind.

Reducing Diets

A severe overweight condition is a big problem. You have to have help from your physician. Here are some suggestions:

A) When you are too round around the middle, follow Dr. Ellis's diet: B_6 and magnesium gluconate, safflower oil, and high protein.
B) If your thighs are too heavy, avoid all sweets for good. Have more gland food such as liver; sprouts; and vitamins E, B_1, and B-complex.
C) If you are too heavy all around, try Gaylord Hauser's Fourteen Day Rejuvenation Diet. Count calories and drink a tea made of chickweed, burdock, and nettle brewed for 20 minutes.
D) When waterlogged, try wheat germ and middlings for one week. Also use vitamins E and C, which act as diuretics and are treasured by many people for this property.

For people who are sensitive to their environment and the negative force fields of others, it is advisable to protect themselves from destruction by putting on some weight. It certainly helps a lot.

Fasting to Achieve Harmonization of the Digestive Tract

Dr. Mayr, of Germany, invented a truly genuine fasting procedure. His theory is that to have health, your digestive tract has to be in good shape. He said that no food, vitamin, or mineral can properly be used in the body unless the digestive tract is functioning well.

Here is his fasting regimen, which should be continued for four to six weeks. One can do it during vacation or in a resort, but many do it while working full time. I must say it is astoundingly easy and unusually effective. Ask your baker to supply you with hard rolls. If you don't have a bakery, make your own. Let these rolls sit for one day until they become ready to cut without crumbling. Again, the rolls should not be too dry, which would interfere with your program. For the success of the fast, it is important that the rolls have the right consistency—not fresh and not too dry. Start your day with a light solution of Epsom salts water. Take one teaspoon Epsom salts in four ounces water and drink slowly. Cut your rolls in small pieces and chew each piece very thoroughly and long, until it is liquefied and becomes sweet. Now, take one teaspoon of milk or buttermilk. Then take the next piece of roll and continue until you are really satisfied. It is amazing how long this meal stays with you. You are not hungry at all until noon, then you do the same thing. Between meals, drink herbal teas such as chamomile, linden blossom, peppermint, or any other tea with a little honey. At night, eat rolled oats blended through a sieve, or wheat prepared the same way, and eat your rolls with sips of milk. Never drink milk alone even when you have some left over in your cup. This would bloat you, and disturb the bacteria you are trying to rebuild in your intestinal tract. Every day, take the juice of one lemon or one orange to supply you with vitamin C and trace elements. After the stool begins to have a golden color and is odorless (about one to two weeks), you add one soft-boiled egg, some butter, cottage cheese, and some creamed soup, but let these be additions to the fundamental roll and milk diet.

Dr. Mayr knows that this regimen is lacking in protein and vitamins, but do not be disturbed by this. A sick digestive tract cannot digest the best food you place in it. It only makes gas, putrefaction, and deposits (because it is so weak). Everything settles in the pockets, curves, and folds of the tract. So first reestablish the proper functioning of the colon, and you will be satisfied with the end result.

Mrs. Clark was 50 years old, but appeared to be much older. Her abdomen was protruding heavily. Her skin looked gray and wrinkled. She had a double chin and her exhaustion was visible and expressed in every movement she made. All her life, she had been on laxatives, sometimes four to six a day, but with very poor results. Mrs. Clark started Dr. Mayr's method in a German clinic and returned to the United States four weeks later a different woman. Gone was the double chin. Gone was the protruding abdomen. No more laxatives. She appeared to be ten years younger. She continued to improve, and by Christmas, her skin was almost wrinkle free.

How does Dr. Mayr's diet work?

a) It reestablishes friendly bacteria.
b) It lubricates every morsel put in the mouth.
c) It relaxes the nerves of the intestinal tract.
d) It takes out accumulated poisons.
e) It harmonizes the intestinal tract.

Dr. Mayr stated that in many people, parts of the in
too fast. Others are spastic, other parts are clogged with
ers work normally. The harmonization of the intestinal tract also ..
expressed in the harmonization of the human individual. From a cranky, sickly, complaining man or woman rises a phoenix of beauty and harmony.

Fasting Replaces Sleep

Whenever you have to miss sleep, drink acidophilus culture. It comes in
pint bottles. Take one-half cup several times a day with very, very little raw
food, just to satisfy your stomach nerves and muscles. Increasingly you will
feel better and better. Whenever you can sleep again, your sleep will be normal in length, and you will wake up refreshed as always. I can verify this
method myself. Sometimes I get carried away and work through my sleeping
hours. Acidophilus replaces my sleep and makes thinking clear.

Revitalizing Diet

After eating a lifetime of wrong food combinations poisoned by chemicals, additives, and no energy, your body rebels. Nothing works any longer.
The eyes give out. Everything hurts. The blood pressure plays escalator (up
and down with every mood). The heart pounds and shortness of breath
begins. In short, you are going to pieces! Now is the time to think of doing
something fundamental, something that will change your life, something that
turns the ship around!

Saturday morning make your decision for one week and two days, and
these will be the best nine days of your life.

7 A.M.	4 oz. sauerkraut juice
	4 oz. tomato juice
8 A.M.	6 to 7 oz. hot lemon juice
9 A.M.	6 to 7 oz. hot vegetable broth
10 A.M.	6 to 7 oz. cool grapefruit juice
11 A.M.	6 to 7 oz. hot vegetable broth
12 NOON	large green salad with dressing of vinegar, sea salt, oil, and spices; cucumber and tomato slices allowed

1 P.M.	6 to 7 oz. cool grapefruit juice
2 P.M.	6 to 7 oz. hot vegetable broth
3 P.M.	6 to 7 oz. cool lemonade
4 P.M.	6 to 7 oz. hot vegetable broth
5 P.M.	6 to 7 oz. cool grapefruit juice
6 P.M.	vegetable salad as at noon
7 P.M.	6 to 7 oz. hot vegetable broth
8 P.M.	yogurt, buttermilk, or juice

If you need a laxative, take it at bedtime. You should have good bowel action. Every third day make the following enema (exception: not when you are a diabetic):

1 quart water and ¾ cup honey—mix well.

In the morning, whenever you have time, cleanse your system with it.

This diet of hot and cold (please, no ice), of salty and sweet (grapefruit juice), stimulates the complete defense mechanism of your body. The tissue lets go of the accumulated waste material. The bowels empty, and the pancreas and liver clean house. The brain starts throwing out the cobwebs, and lymph and blood are rejuvenated.

I suggest you take a little cabin somewhere away from temptation and the suggestions of your friends and enjoy the return of your health.

Clean Your Lymphatic System

Try the following recipe:

1 pint white grapefruit juice
1 pint freshly squeezed orange juice
1 pint grape juice
1 pint water with the juice of three limes
1 pint water with the juice of two lemons
1 pint frozen pineapple juice, diluted
1 pint papaya juice, diluted
12 eggs (whole)
6 egg yolks

frozen raspberries or strawberries add a delicious flavor
beat eggs and mix into fruit juice mixture

This is one day's supply. If you are hungry, add one kind of fresh fruit. For lunch, green salad and/or sprouts with raw almond dressing. For supper, green salad and/or sprouts with raw almond dressing and one steamed vegetable.

Apple Juice Diet

I have a book from the seventeenth century in which an old physician from Austria reveals his secrets. One of them is the apple juice diet. This diet is greatly used among health-minded people to detoxify the liver and gall-bladder. I recommend it to everyone very highly.

First Day

8 A.M.	1 glass (8 oz.) apple juice
10 A.M.	2 glasses (16 oz.) apple juice
12 NOON	2 glasses (16 oz.) apple juice
2 P.M.	2 glasses (16 oz.) apple juice
4 P.M.	2 glasses (16 oz.) apple juice
6 P.M.	2 glasses (16 oz.) apple juice
8 P.M.	2 glasses (16 oz.) apple juice

Juice should be natural, without chemicals. No food is to be taken this day.

Second Day

Follow the same procedure as the first day. No food this day either. At bedtime, take four ounces of olive oil. You may wash the olive oil down with hot lemon juice or hot apple juice.

As a rule, this diet starts to work around 4 A.M. In the fecal matter, you will find little green pebbles. They may be the size of a pinhead, or they may be as big as a bird egg. Many times it all looks like green mud. In any case, the old stagnant bile becomes dissolved and liquefied through the malic acid of the apple juice, which should be sugar and chemical free, and the oil moves the whole thing.

Dr. Adolphus Hohensee has been using this diet on thousands of his students all over America. In Europe, it is practiced in health spas and hospitals with equal results. It reestablishes the normal function of the liver. This diet "frees the liver-gallbladder trace from the old bile and debris, which we call stones!"

The old American Indian recipe for liver trouble is chaparral tea and/or fringe tree bark. Chaparral is a creosote bush from the desert and tastes very nasty. Mayo Clinic became interested in this herb and is doing research at the present time. Some manufacturers make chaparral in tablet form, and it is available in health food stores and sometimes drugstores.

All liver teas are bitter. It is as if nature wants to heal bitter gall with bitter teas. Dandelion leaves and root, gentian and fringe tree are relief to an ailing liver. These herbs were in use for centuries, and they are still good today.

Liver Rejuvenating Recipes

I found the following recipe in an old book used in 1802 by Dr. Selig of Austria. It sounded so good that I tried it and found it truly excellent.

1 teaspoon dandelion root
1 teaspoon angelica or arnica
1 teaspoon wormwood
1 teaspoon gentian

Boil in two cups water, simmer, and strain. Add two quarts apple juice and 4 ounces freshly squeezed lemon juice and drink this in small portions during the day. Do this for two to three days and repeat as needed once a month. Take only stewed fruit and apple juice on these days.

Also for the liver:
Wash one average-size grapefruit and cut in small pieces. Add one and one-half quarts water and boil for 15 minutes. Strain off the liquid and sweeten with honey. Drink six ounces once a day.

Part III

HEALTH ISSUES AND HEALING REMEDIES

Chapter Fifteen

❁

HOME REMEDIES

The following chart lists health concerns and the corresponding vitamins, minerals, and home remedies that will correct the problem. If not already in your kitchen, many of these homeopathic remedies, teas, and herbs can be found in your local health food store.

HEALTH ISSUE REMEDIES

	Vitamins/ Minerals	Spices/Herbs/ Kitchen Aids
Abdomen: distended without nausea		Nutmeg: ½ tsp. in hot water
Abdominal tenderness		Linden flower tea 12-herb tincture formula[1]: Rub on navel.
Absence of all moral restraint		Cashew nut (*Anacardium occidentale*)
Achilles tendon pain		St. Ignatius's bean (*Ignatia amara*) (homeopathic)

[1] The herbs include apple tree bark, calamus root, burdock root, pimpernel root, angelica root, cherry bark, rhubarb root, gentian root, aloes, cascara sagrada bark, nutmeg, and myrrh.

HEALTH ISSUE	REMEDIES	
	Vitamins/ Minerals	Spices/Herbs/ Kitchen Aids
Acid indigestion	B_1, B_2, minerals from raw potatoes	Yarrow tea: Drink ½ cup two times daily. Raw potatoes
Acid stomach	B-complex, niacin	
Acidosis (acid dyspepsia)	B_1, minerals from raw potatoes	Raw potato: Eat a piece before each meal.
Acne (see also Boils and pimples; Pimples)	A, C, B_6 (young people) A, C, B_2, E (common)	For facial acne: Try homeopathic *Bellis perennis* (daisy). Dandelion, nettle, strawberry leaves: Single or together as tea. Charcoal tablets: Take two before each meal daily. Buttermilk and honey: Boil buttermilk; when thickened, add honey so it becomes a thick cream. Apply wherever needed. Walnut leaves Avoid all chocolate.
Adrenal gland	C, B-complex, pantothenic acid, sodium PABA: 2 tablets	Alfalfa Seeds: Take 1 tbl. seeds. Licorice root: Make tea or chew the root. Dates and sunflower seed drink. Protein: More needed.
Aging: preventing (see also Weakness)		12-herb tincture formula[1]; Lavender; Sage; Thyme

[1] The herbs include apple tree bark, calamus root, burdock root, pimpernel root, angelica root, cherry bark, rhubarb root, gentian root, aloes, cascara sagrada bark, nutmeg, and myrrh.

HEALTH ISSUE — REMEDIES

	Vitamins/ Minerals	Spices/Herbs/ Kitchen Aids
Aging: preventing (cont.)		Sarsaparilla root, dried: Bring 1 tsp. of sarsaparilla root and 1 cup of cold water to a boil and then turn down and simmer for 5 minutes. Drink 6 ozs. twice daily. Whey: Premature aging is a mineral deficiency. Whey has lots of minerals. It will keep muscles young, joints moveable, and ligaments elastic.
Alcohol (drinking too much)	B_1: 100 mg. 3 times daily	Cucumber (enzyme called erepsin): Reduces the alcohol's intoxicating effect. Honey: Removes alcohol from the blood extra fast.
Alcoholism (candida encased in liver)	Alcoholics suffer from severe vitamin C, B, and zinc deficiencies. B-complex, B_1, B_{12}, E, choline, inositol, pantothenic acid, niacin	Sometimes there are parasites in the pancreas; take a specific remedy to help. Chromium and vanadium mixed together: Take 1 tsp. twice daily to reduce the desire for alcohol. Take 1 tbl. Epsom salts in the morning and 1 tbl. at night. The herb ginkgo biloba is a help for alcohol cravings. Thyme tea: Helps stop the desire.
Alkali reserve (loss of)	B_1	Apple cider vinegar: Take 2 tsps. in 1 cup of water with honey.

HEALTH ISSUE	REMEDIES	
	Vitamins/ Minerals	Spices/Herbs/ Kitchen Aids
Allergen	B, C, E	Watercress: It's an antiallergen full of vitamins E, B, and C. Used to decorate salads, sandwiches, and sauces. When eaten by itself, give only small portions since it's potent.
Allergic to wool	Magnesium	
Allergies (general)	A, G, B$_6$, B$_{12}$, E, pantothenic acid, L-histidine	Wild plum bark syrup Sage: Use on a piece of buttered whole-grain bread (rye or wheat). Orange rind or peelings mixed in a tea: Relieves stuffed up nose and clogged air passages, and healthful sleep results. Banana: For energy and nerves; hinders allergies. Honey: To relieve symptoms, you should use honey from your own neighborhood. It can act as an antihistamine. To cleanse lymphatic system: Every ½ hour drink 4 oz. pure water. Do this for 2 days. Then make a vegetable broth and drink on the hour 6 oz. broth, and on the ½ hour 4 oz. water. All allergies have two factors in common: chemical poison and parasites. See a physician to find your parasites.

<small>HEALTH ISSUE</small> <small>REMEDIES</small>

	Vitamins/ Minerals	Spices/Herbs/ Kitchen Aids
Always cold	Iodine	
Amoeba		Garlic: Take 3 to 6 capsules daily. Jasmine tea: Take 1 cup 3 times daily. Papaya leaf: Eat one daily to protect. *Ipecacuanha* (homeopathic)
Amoebic dysentery		*Ipecacuanha* (homeopathic)
Anemia (see also Spleen)	A, B_2, B_6, B_{12} Copper, iron	Manukka raisins, molasses: Contain extra minerals. Beet juice and yellow dock contain iron. Eggplant: Reduces enlarged spleen and increases red blood corpuscles and hemoglobin. Grape juice, blackstrap molasses: 2 tsps. molasses in 1 glass grape juice. Grape juice: 1 glass juice and 1 egg yolk. Lentils contain protein supplies and iron of the best quality. Pumpkin seeds: Chew well. Raisins and grapefruit: 2 ozs. dark raisins 3 times daily for 1 day; ½ grapefruit twice daily second day; alternate for 3 weeks.

HEALTH ISSUE   REMEDIES

	Vitamins/ Minerals	Spices/Herbs/ Kitchen Aids
Anemia (cont.)		Spinach: Blood builder; raw is best. Wine: ½ glass red wine, ½ glass water, 2 egg yolks.
Anger (over little things)	Sodium	
Angina pectoris		Apple cider vinegar: Heat apple cider vinegar. Wet a Turkish towel with warm vinegar. Apply to the back and chest of angina sufferer until help arrives.
Ankles, pain		St. John's wort (*Hypericum perforatum*) (homeopathic)
Ankles and feet (pain)		Pokeroot tea: Drink two cups daily and soak feet.
Ankles, pain in joints		Potato peelings: Simmer one handful in 2 cups of water for 15 minutes. Strain and take 2 tbls. in 1 glass of water 4 times daily for 14 days. After several days, legs and ankles should be more normal size.
Ankles, weak		Scotch pine tea: Make a strong tea and wrap compresses around ankles.

Health Issue	Remedies	
	Vitamins/ Minerals	Spices/Herbs/ Kitchen Aids
Anorexia Nervosa (refusal to eat, causing severe weight loss)	Possible zinc deficiency	Good sources of zinc: lean meat, poultry, fish, shellfish, oatmeal, whole wheat bread, peas, lima beans, egg yolks, brewer's yeast, wheat germ, milk, and yogurt. Cloves help to stimulate the appetite, making it easier to recover. Rub your earlobes several times a day.
Antibiotic		Avocado seeds: Pound seeds and make tea.
Antifat		Bladderwrack: Take in tablet form.
Antiseptic		Lemon: Use externally on sores, corns, and dandruff. Gargle with it. Drink plenty when fever hits.
Antispasmodic		Balm leaf tea: 1 cup as needed. Caraway: Improves appetite, subsides gastric distention, takes out phlegm, and useful for stomach disorders. Cinquefoil tea: Drink ½ cup as needed. Skullcap
Anti-tobacco		Apple: detoxifying

HEALTH ISSUE   REMEDIES

	Vitamins/ Minerals	Spices/Herbs/ Kitchen Aids
Anti-tumor		Garlic: Natural antibiotic; has M-rays to search out harmful agents.
Anus, biting		Peony (*Paeonia officinalis*) tea
Anus, burning		Blue flag (*Iris versicolor*) tea
Anus, itching (see also Liver)		Ground ivy tea: Take 1 cup a day.
Anus, painful		Ginger tea: Drink ½ cup 3 times a day.
Anxiety	Lack of chromium and magnesium	Borage and thyme tea.
Apathy		Saw Palmetto (*Sabal serrulata*) (homeopathic)
Appearance, dull	Iodine	
Appetite, loss of	B_6, B_{12}	Apples help regain appetite. Alfalfa in small amounts creates sound appetite and improves digestion. Caraway and eggplant improve appetite. Homeopathic: Dandelion (*Taraxacum officinale*)
Appetite, loss of in children		Cranberry juice or sauce

HEALTH ISSUE | REMEDIES

Health Issue	Vitamins/ Minerals	Spices/Herbs/ Kitchen Aids
Arches, fallen		Comfrey root tincture: Apply overnight on soles of feet.
Arm-shoulder syndrome (pain)	B-complex, B_{12}, folic acid	
Arms (nodules in)		Homeopathic: *Hippozaurium* helps.
Arms (pain in upper left)		Watch the heart. Sometimes the muscle in the arms hurt because of arsenic poisoning in the muscles.
Arteries		Yogurt and applesauce: 1 dish daily to keep arteries clean. Aloe vera aids in assimilation, circulation, and elimination.
Arteriosclerosis (hardening of arteries)	A, B_{12}, E	Apple tree bark tea Parsley: Keeps arteries clear. Combine: Brussels sprouts, alfalfa, garlic, vitamin F, whey, violet, hyssop, clover; eat 4 cups per day. Distilled water, lecithin Indian remedy: Tea of sassafras. Also, take ½ tsp. cream of tartar, twice weekly. A combination of hawthorn berries, *Equisetum* concentrate, vit-amin C, taurine, arginine,

HEALTH ISSUE	REMEDIES	
	Vitamins/ Minerals	Spices/Herbs/ Kitchen Aids
Arteriosclerosis (cont.)		chromium picolinate, and selenium, along with aloe vera gel
Arthritis	A, B-complex, B_1, B_{15}, D, E Trace minerals from alfalfa seeds When diet is too alkaline: Add calcium, protein from pumpkin seeds, and take okra tablets for extra minerals.	Apple cider vinegar, honey, water: Combine 2 tsps. each vinegar and honey in 8 ozs. of water. Take 3 times daily with meals. Avocado seed: Pound, make strong tea, and apply to skin. Celery, parsley, and celeriac: Eat celery and parsley every day or juice them and eat celeriac. Five foods: Black cherry juice; peanut oil, 2 tbls.; alfalfa seeds, juice, or tablets; celeriac or celery root; liquid rice B-complex. Flaxseed: Can be used externally or internally. Garlic: Crush, spread in cloth like butter on bread. Wrap poultice around arthritic joint 2 to 12 hours, which will raise a large blister full of water. This will break and run out, drawing the disease out of the joint. Heal the burn with aloe vera juice and see amazing results.

HEALTH ISSUE REMEDIES

	Vitamins/ Minerals	Spices/Herbs/ Kitchen Aids
Arthritis (cont.)		Lemon, orange, grapefruit: Grate 1 lemon, 1 orange, 1 grapefruit. Add 2 tsps. cream of tartar, 2 tbls. Epsom salts, 1 quart water. Drink 2 ozs. 3 times daily.
		Oil of wintergreen: Rub on joints; also, rub kerosene on joints.
		Eat strawberries, cranberries, asparagus, and Swiss chard.
		Whey: Mix 2 tbls. with 1 tbl. lecithin and 8 tbls. of vegetable broth. Take 3 times daily for several months.
		Brown paper: Make layers, sew between two layers of flannel, and use as a bed covering. The DMSO pine residue relieves pain and heals.
		Willow bark: Make tea.
Arthritis, deformation of hands and feet		Comfrey root: Make and apply warm compresses.
		Cabbage leaf: Heat and apply overnight.
Arthritis, prone to	Phosphorus	
Asthma	A, C, B-complex, choline, inositol, lecithin, E	Anise tea
		Cinnamon; Wild cherry bark
		Elecampane and quebracho: Gallbladder flush.

HEALTH ISSUE	REMEDIES	
	Vitamins/ Minerals	Spices/Herbs/ Kitchen Aids
Asthma (cont.)		Thyme powder mixed with honey. Dosage: 1 tsp. every hour.
		Wild plum bark: Make syrup and take 1 tbl. 4 times daily. Make a pillow and sleep with it. Good for hay fever, too.
		Wormwood: Boil in apple juice.
		Lemon juice: Take 2 tbls. before each meal.
		Radish and honey: Grate black radish; add honey. Before going to bed take 1 tsp. of the mixture.
		Go on a ½ day fast. The time you don't eat, take 2 quarts of water, soak green pineapples in it, and let sit for 2 hours. Drink from that fluid for the other half of the day (all you want). Do this for 10 to 14 days.
		Red onion (raw) juice mixed with raw sugar. Dosage: 1 tsp. every hour.
		Sunflower seeds: Combine 1 quart sunflower seeds in ½ gallon water; boil down to 1 quart of water. Strain, add 1 pint honey, and boil down to a syrup.
		Give 1 tsp. 3 times daily.
		Homeopathic remedy for adults: yerba santa (*Eriodictyon glutinosum*).

HEALTH ISSUE	REMEDIES	
	Vitamins/ Minerals	Spices/Herbs/ Kitchen Aids
Asthma attack		Cranberry juice concentrate: One tsp. can stop an attack. To make your own: Boil 1 pint water and 1 pound cranberries until done, then refrigerate. Dosage: 1 tsp. Put hands in hot water.
Asthma, in children		*Thuja occidentalis* (homeopathic)
Asthma, through nervousness		Dandelion root-and-leaves tea
Asthma, upon sleeping		Spikenard tea: Take 1 tsp. twice daily.
Asthma, without anxiety		Ginger Wild plum bark, wild cherry bark: 1 tsp. to 1 cup of tea.
Astigmatism (myopic) (see also Myopic Astigmatism)		Tiger lily (*Lilium tigrinum*) (homeopathic)
Athlete's foot	A	Bathe feet in rosehips tea or lemon juice or follow suggestions on Clorox bottle. Spinach seed and onion seed: Simmer 2 tbls. of the seeds in 1 quart of water for ½ hour; then soak feet in the water. Quaw bark tincture: Apply externally.

HEALTH ISSUE	REMEDIES	
	Vitamins/ Minerals	Spices/Herbs/ Kitchen Aids
Attention Deficit Disorder (ADD)	B₁ supplement will help.	A tea combination of rosemary, blue vervain, and calamus heals the trauma. Homeopathic: *Plumbum metallicum* clears the lead poisoning (a possible cause of ADD). A homeopathic remedy specific to ADD helps eliminate poisons.
Aura cleanser		Rose petals, cyani flowers, yarrow: Combine and brew; steep, strain, and add to bathwater.
Autism	Calcium, magnesium, vitamin B₆, and chromium for the hypoglycemia	A specific remedy for parasites in the pancreas. Avoid sugar and food allergens.
Aversion to darkness	Calcium fluoride	
Aversion to water		Homeopathic: Thorn apple (*Stramonium*) A lack of amino acids will cause an aversion; also, a lack of protein.
Babies, healthy		Squaw vine Milk: Mama's is best; goat's milk, next best. Ripe banana and ripe coconut ground and squeezed are very good.

HEALTH ISSUE	REMEDIES	
	Vitamins/ Minerals	Spices/Herbs/ Kitchen Aids
Backache, affecting hips and sacrum (walking stooped)		Horse chestnut
Backache, in children		Alfalfa seed, dill seed
Backache, lumbar region		Pokeroot tea: Simmer root; 2 cups daily.
Backward children		Alfalfa seed tea Dill: Add to food as seasoning. Bran: pour 8 ozs. of boiling water over 1 tbl. bran. Add honey to taste and give to children, invalids, and mentally disturbed people.
Bacterial infection		Cabbage: It's anti-inflammatory, antibacterial, and encourages new cell growth. Onions: Absorb bacteria; can be used to help disinfect sickroom. Goldenseal root (*Hydrastis canadensis*) (homeopathic) Black pepper: Kills bacteria and can be used as a food preservative. Garlic; Cinnamon; Fiber in whole-grain foods
Bad breath (see also Breath, bad)	Possible zinc deficiency	Sometimes a disturbed function of the gallbladder or liver or both. May also be a sign of major gum disease.

HEALTH ISSUE	REMEDIES	
	Vitamins/ Minerals	Spices/Herbs/ Kitchen Aids
Bad breath (cont.)		Try sipping thyme tea or chewing on dill seeds to freshen breath. Caraway seed and anise seed, mixed together. Homeopathic: *Arsenicum album; Baptisia tinctoria*
Baldness	PABA, biotin, folic acid, inositol	
Bedsores	C, E, copper	
Bed-wetting	B_1, B-complex, E, magnesium	Avoid sugar, simple sugars, and allergenic foods. Bistort tea, equisetum tea, violet leaf tea: Serve no later than 4 hours before bedtime. Cinnamon: Helps prevent bed-wetting and also promotes sleep. Homeopathic: Cuttlefish (*Sepia*); *Calcerea phosphorica*
Bee sting (In the mouth or throat: this is a serious accident.)		Salt: Take 1 tsp. of salt and put in the mouth at once. It has prevented many from strangling to death. Onion: Rub raw onion on the area.
Belching		Papaya tablets have an enzyme that will prevent belching. Saw palmetto tea

HEALTH ISSUE	REMEDIES	
	Vitamins/ Minerals	Spices/Herbs/ Kitchen Aids
Belching (cont.)		Try massaging earlobes. Avoid carbonated beverages, eat slowly, avoid chewing gum, and avoid foods with high air content.
Bile, duct sluggish		Mugwort: Take ½ cup tea, a strong herb. Celandine (*Chelidonium majus*) tea: ½ cup before meals. Artichoke: Brings a clear urine and increases the flow of bile. It is also claimed that it keeps the arteries smooth and a person free from weak digestion. Useful for albumin in the urine and jaundice. Soup: Small bowl at the beginning of meal is stimulating to the bile.
Bile, increase		Black garden radish: Eat 1 before meals.
Birthmarks		Castor oil: Apply for several months.
Bites (see also Insect Bites; Mosquito bites)		Dog or cat bite: Assess damage to determine if you need medical attention. Then thoroughly wash the wound with soap and water. Continue washing for 5 full minutes. Do not shy away from a tetanus shot. Take Homeopathic Thuja afterwards.

HEALTH ISSUE   REMEDIES

	Vitamins/ Minerals	Spices/Herbs/ Kitchen Aids
Bites (cont.)		Rattlesnake bite: Wet some salt and wrap the bitten arm or leg in a salt pack, making sure the bite gets an extra dose of salt. Then, RUSH to your physician. Poisonous Spider: Consult physician. Use the homeopathic Glondirine as well.
Bitter taste in mouth	Potassium	
Blackheads	A	Cucumber: Cut a piece and rub over face. Also, cover face with cucumber peelings, the cut side to the skin. Strawberries: Rub fresh berries over face. Wash face with hot water, and then sprinkle with cold water. Use soap and water, lathering freely; dry, rinse thoroughly. Afterwards, sponge with witch hazel. Repeat daily.
Bladder	A, B_6, magnesium	
Bladder, hemorrhage		Peach tree bark tea: Drink 3 cups daily. Comfrey root: Drink 3 cups daily.

HEALTH ISSUE | REMEDIES

Health Issue	Vitamins/ Minerals	Spices/Herbs/ Kitchen Aids
Bladder, infection	A, B$_6$, C, E Trace minerals from uva ursi	Collinsonia root tea Cranberry juice (drink plenty) Pomegranate: Juice it and mix ½ cup with ½ cup water, and sip it. It is even better as a fruit eaten twice a day. Take a wool blanket and spread on your bed. Place a cotton sheet over it, and sleep on it. (Will also help with kidney problems.)
Bladder, pain		Marshmallow root: If due to a cold, take 1 tbl. marshmallow root in 1 cup water. Drink hot. Pomegranate: As a juice, ½ cup with ½ cup water. Better as fruit; eat one twice a day.
Bladder, stones		Carrot leaves, parsley tea: 1 quart a day for 3 days; then just 2 cups a day for 2 weeks.
Bladder, weak		Pumpkin seed: Take 1 tsp. 3 times daily or more if desired. Chickpea
Bleeding, bowels		Cinnamon tea: Take ½ cup 4 times daily.
Bleeding, cuts		Cover the cut with unglazed brown paper wetted with vinegar.

HEALTH ISSUE	REMEDIES	
	Vitamins/ Minerals	Spices/Herbs/ Kitchen Aids
Bleeding, female (see Female, bleeding)		
Bleeding, gums (see also Gum disease)	C, E, P, K₂ Chromium	Black pepper: Freshly ground, it's loaded with chromium, which is needed for proper functioning of the pancreas and heart. Lemons: Wash and cut 6 lemons in little pieces. Cover with 1½ quarts of water and bring to a boil. Turn off heat and let sit for 25 minutes. Strain and set aside until cool. Take 6 ozs. 2 times daily for 10 days. In case of bleeding gums, hold juice in your mouth, also. Papaya seeds: Chew 1 tsp. papaya seeds 4 times daily and spit out after chewing thoroughly.
Bleeding, intestinal		Shepherd's purse tea: Drink 1 cup twice a day.
Bleeding, tooth (after extraction)		Black tea: Moisten one tea bag with warm water and apply to tooth.
Blisters		Homeopathic: Buttercup (*Ranunculus bulbosus*) for blisters in the palm of your hand. Sage: Eat or make tea and drink for blisters in the mouth.

Health Issue	Remedies	
	Vitamins/ Minerals	Spices/Herbs/ Kitchen Aids
Blisters (cont.)		Arnica and violet tea: Hold in mouth and drink (for blisters in the mouth).
Bloatedness		Caraway and fennel: Take equal parts, grind seeds in blender. Sage with peppermint: Make tea. Fennel: 1 tsp. fennel. Bring to a boil in 8 ozs. of water. Simmer 10 minutes. Strain 1 to 2 cups for adults; children ½ cup. Anise: Make a very diluted tea and give a few drops as needed. Gentian tea: Use ½ to 1 cup a day.
Blood, builders	B_6	Egg yolk: Mix with some concord grape juice. Terrific blood builder. Apricots: Eat two dried, twice daily, or soak and blend them. Blackstrap molasses: Take 2 to 4 tsps. daily. Beet and grape juice: Combine 1 part red beet juice, 2 parts dark grape juice. Take 2 tbls. 3 times daily. Carrots, watermelon seed, bananas: All blood builders. Red clover tea

HEALTH ISSUE   REMEDIES

	Vitamins/ Minerals	Spices/Herbs/ Kitchen Aids
Blood, cleanser		Lemon juice, honey, and water: Take 6 ozs. every 2 hours. Take 1 tsp. sanicle to 1 cup of boiling water. Take 5 parts red clover and 1 part chaparral: Make tea and drink 2 cups daily. Take 1 tsp. sassafras tea to a cup of boiling water (strong cleanser). Take 1 tsp. sheep sorrel to 1 cup of boiling water (strong cleanser).
Blood, poisoning		Cranberries: Boil 1 quart cranberry juice with 8 cloves and 1 tsp. cinnamon. Add 1 quart of water and drink this in a day.
Blood pressure	B_{12}, B-complex, lecithin, garlic for elasticity of the vessels	Parsley: Make parsley tea and also add parsley to salads and soups. Parsley, celery, garlic: Eat plenty of parsley and add garlic and celery. Or buy a juicer, juice the vegetables, and drink 6 ozs. twice daily. Apples: Eat two a day. Turnip tops: Boil turnip tops as you would spinach. Eaten with rice once every day lowers blood pressure.

HEALTH ISSUE REMEDIES

	Vitamins/ Minerals	Spices/Herbs/ Kitchen Aids
Blood pressure (cont.)		Watermelon seeds: Dilate the blood vessels, lower pressure, and improve kidney function.
		Homeopathic: Wild indigo (*Baptisia tinctoria*), Hawthorn (*Crataegus oxycantha*), Cone flower (*Echinacea angustifolia*)
Blood pressure, high (see also High blood pressure)	B₁, B-complex, lecithin, garlic for elasticity of vessels, potassium	Oranges and lemons: 3 oranges, 2 lemons. Cut into pieces. Boil in 1 quart of water for 15 minutes. Then add 2 tbls. of honey. Boil another 10 minutes. Strain and drink 6 ozs., 3 times daily, before meals (not for diabetics).
		Mistletoe and angelica: Combine 2 tsps. of each in 1 quart water; bring to a boil and drink 2 to 3 cups a day.
		Garlic regulates blood pressure.
		Peas and beans (for potassium)
		Homeopathic: *Uranium nitricum.*
Blood pressure, low	B₁, B₆, B-complex Copper, iron, niacin	Cayenne: Add to your food.
		Apricots: Mix with dark raisins. Eat 2 tbls., 3 times daily.
		Protein
		Homeopathic: *Cactus grandiflorus*

HEALTH ISSUE	REMEDIES	
	Vitamins/ Minerals	Spices/Herbs/ Kitchen Aids
Blood, purifier		Purifying foods: Beets, carrots, cranberries, cucumbers, strawberry leaves for skin Hyssop tea
Blood, thinners		Rosemary and red clover: Red clover tea from leaves; red clover tea from seeds (stronger).
Blood, toxins		Cranberries: Boil 1 quart cranberry juice with 8 cloves and 1 tsp. cinnamon. Add 1 quart of water and drink this in a day.
Blurred vision	B_6	
Body odor	Zinc, calcium/magnesium, plant-derived colloidal minerals	Chlorophyll: Everything green has chlorophyll. Take plenty of green drinks or buy liquid chlorophyll to combat body odor. Parsley contains chlorophyll. Drink tomato juice daily. Lots of green, leafy vegetables; alfalfa
Boils	A, C, bioflavonoids, E	Onions: Put onion poultice over a boil to bring it to a head. Tomato: Cut the stem out of a ripe tomato; turn tomato over the boil to bring it to a head. (Indian remedy)

HEALTH ISSUE   REMEDIES

	Vitamins/ Minerals	Spices/Herbs/ Kitchen Aids
Boils (cont.)		Garden sage and corn-meal: Use as a poultice. Flaxseed poultice See your physician.
Boils and pimples		Nutmeg: Combine ⅓ tsp. nutmeg (freshly ground), 1 tsp. honey, and 4 to 5 ozs. hot water. Drink 3 mornings in a row. Don't drink it for 3 days. Repeat nine times.
Bones, brittle	B-complex, B_{12}, C, E Calcium (bonemeal), potassium	Cabbage builds bones. Bananas (potassium) keep bones healthy.
Bones, broken		Comfrey root Wild geranium tea Take an orange towel and sleep on it. Also, use it when bones are healed but still give trouble.
Bones, crackle when walking	Manganese	
Bones, marrow		Yarrow tea (strengthener)
Bones, pain		Comfrey root tea Comfrey root tincture
Bones, tendon and muscle injuries		Comfrey root compresses Arnica root is best.

HEALTH ISSUE | REMEDIES

Health Issue	Vitamins/ Minerals	Spices/Herbs/ Kitchen Aids
Bones, Coxsackie virus		A specific homeopathic remedy for Coxsackie.
Bones, weak		Fenugreek seed: Take in tablet or capsule form.
Booster (see also Pep drink)		Chia seed, sunflower seed, sesame seed, flax-seed: Mix equal portions and soak 1 tbl. overnight in ½ glass of water. Next morning, add ½ glass juice or more. Drink this once a day for energy.
Botulism		Apple cider vinegar: 2 tsps. in 7 ozs. of warm water and sip slowly. For children, add honey.
Bowels		Alfalfa helps them move. Black pepper tea will help running bowels. Barley is excellent food for children suffering from inflammation of the bowels.
Bowels, bleeding		Cinnamon bark tea: ½ cup 4 times a day will heal all bleeding bowels. Or chew on cinnamon bark until you can visit your physician.
Bowels, cleansing		Flaxseed: Gently simmer for about ½ hour, then let stand where it will remain hot for 1 or 2 hours longer.

HEALTH ISSUE   REMEDIES

	Vitamins/ Minerals	Spices/Herbs/ Kitchen Aids
Bowels, cleansing (cont.)		Combine 2 tbls. in 2 cups of boiling water; let it boil down to 1 cup. Add sugar to taste. Add the juice of ½ lemon if you want. Drink the whole cupful at bedtime and swallow all the seeds. Take about once a week, every 4 days, or more often if needed. It is harmless. Molasses and lemon: When there is lots of gas present, combine 1 tbl. molasses, the juice of 1 lemon, and 1 quart of hot water. Always check for protozoa and worms.
Bowels, dropped		Prickly pear
Brain, food	B_{12}, folic acid, gotu kola to strengthen concentration	Combine 1 lb. sunflower seeds, ¼ lb. almonds, 1 lb. wheat; grind up and eat 2 heaping tbls. a day. Cardamom is an eye and brain food. Brain cocktail: Combine 1 cup barley, 1 cup coconut juice, 1 tbl. lecithin. Honey if desired. Coconut: Eat the meat and drink the milk. Leeks: Cut, boil, and use in soups or salads.

HEALTH ISSUE	REMEDIES	
	Vitamins/ Minerals	Spices/Herbs/ Kitchen Aids
Brain, food (cont.)		Dried apple peelings made into tea are full of silicon, which will strengthen the brain.
		Almonds; almond oil: Only 1 tsp. daily will improve memory.
		Oats help memory.
		Cloves in tea will heighten memory.
		Sage: Put on a slice of lightly buttered rye bread.
		Eyebright in capsules or tablets strengthen memory.
		Take 2 mustard seeds to improve memory.
		Take hawthorn tablets or as tea to combat mental dullness.
		Lemon balm to promote youth and strengthen the brain.
		Take Dulcamara or purple cone flower to clear up mental confusion.
		Basil: Eat it or wash your hands, arms, and face with basil tea.
		Homeopathic: Honey bee (Apis mellifica)
Brain, tumor		Tofu: Shave head, apply tofu over head, and change the compress when tofu gets yellow.

HEALTH ISSUE   REMEDIES

	Vitamins/ Minerals	Spices/Herbs/ Kitchen Aids
Brain, tumor (cont.)		Tomato: Use raw crushed tomato in a cheesecloth poultice.
Breast, caked and sore		Carrots: Grate raw carrots and apply to hardened and sore breast.
Breast, knots in		Laurel leaves: Simmer in oil and apply to breast gently without pressure. Carrots: Grate and make a poultice over breast.
Breast, lumps or pain		Bag balm available at veterinary supply house.
Breast, sticky pain in left		Myrtle tea
Breath, bad (foul odor) (see also Bad breath)	Sodium	
Breath, shortness of		Black tea: A cup of black tea often relieves breathing difficulty until you find a doctor's help. Red onion juice: Bring to a boil, add honey, simmer for 15 minutes. Take 1 tsp. every hour. One tbl. raw onion juice with 1 tsp. sugar.
Bright's disease (kidney trouble) (see also Kidneys, catarrhal)		Watermelon seed: For 2 days eat nothing but watermelon. Eat always by itself.

HEALTH ISSUE   REMEDIES

	Vitamins/ Minerals	Spices/Herbs/ Kitchen Aids
Bromide poison (or narcotic poisoning)		Coffee: Give strong coffee by mouth or enema when someone has taken an overdose of bromide. One cup every hour. When the victim is in a stupor, give coffee enema every half hour.
Bronchitis		Flaxseed: To 1 pint of flaxseed tea, add the juice of 2 lemons, and 3 tbls. honey. Take 1 tsp. every half hour until relieved. Myrtle leaves: Contain Myrtal, an active antiseptic. Use as a tea. White hellebore: For elderly with bronchitis. Myrrh: Use in chest rubs for congestion. Helpful herbs: Daffodil, lugworm, plantain. Take Echinacea, either as tea or in capsule form. 12-herb tincture formula[1]
Bronchitis, prone to	Phosphorus	
Brown spots on skin	Calcium fluoride	
Bruises	C, bioflavonoids, pantothenic acid, K_2, rutin	Chestnut leaves or alfalfa provide K_2. Crushed peach leaves applied as a poultice.

[1] The herbs include apple tree bark, calamus root, burdock root, pimpernel root, angelica root, cherry bark, rhubarb root, gentian root, aloes, cascara sagrada bark, nutmeg, and myrrh.

Health Issue	Remedies	
	Vitamins/ Minerals	Spices/Herbs/ Kitchen Aids
Bruises (cont.)		Solomon's seal or daisy tea poultices. Apply a hot milk and crushed seed (fenugreek) poultice.
Burning, alimentary canal		Blue flag (*Iris versicolor*)
Burning, feet	B_6, B-complex, pantothenic acid, E, copper, iron	Tobacco: Moisten tobacco and slap over bruise. It will burn, but when the burn stops, you can continue to work.
Burning, pains	B_{12}	Cayenne pepper
Burning, sensation in body and limbs	B_{12}, manganese	
Burning, skin with itching		Buttercup (*Ranunculus bulbosus*) (homeopathic)
Burns	C, E	Aloe vera: Apply to burns. Cold water: Place under cold water until all pain is gone. (For minor burns; if serious, begin cold water treatment and call for medical help at once.) Some dip a burn in cold fresh cream if available. Black Tea Egg white: Slightly beaten and applied to first- and second-degree burns will take away pain.

HEALTH ISSUE   REMEDIES

	Vitamins/ Minerals	Spices/Herbs/ Kitchen Aids
Bursitis	Take 2 parts magnesium and 1 part calcium.	Homeopathic: *Arsenicum album* See a chiropractor.
Calcium (need more)		Broccoli contains more available calcium than milk or other sources. Cauliflower: A very good calcium supplier.
Calluses and corns	A, C	Lemon and castor oil Take a piece of lemon and tie over corns overnight. Repeat with a new lemon every night. Rub peppermint oil on calluses. Soak feet in very warm water for 5 minutes. Then buff with pumice to remove dead skin. Homeopathic: Buttercup (*Ranunculus bulbosus*) (for corns)
Cancer		Concord grape juice: Every morning for 6 weeks, drink 1 quart of juice from the time you wake up until noon, with no other food. After noon, eat normally. Emphasize almonds, asparagus, and other fruits and vegetables, with no heavy protein after 2 P.M. Used in Europe with outstanding results.

HEALTH ISSUE	REMEDIES	
	Vitamins/ Minerals	Spices/Herbs/ Kitchen Aids
Cancer (cont.)		Orange peelings: Dried, boiled; use for cancer patients having pain, particularly if cancer is in mouth or tongue. Cabbage: Valuable for its healing properties.
Cancer (prevention)	Iodine (from asparagus) may be helpful in preventing cancer and other cell-destroying diseases.	Garlic: Found to block the formation of colon cancer and may prevent other types. Cabbage: Contains ingredients that prevent cancer. Important dietary addition. Asparagus: Contains substances that assist body in normal cell formation. Antioxidants protecting against cancer: apricots, cantaloupe, carrots, citrus fruits, kale, parsley, spinach, sweet potatoes, turnip greens, winter squash, yams. Broccoli, cucumber, eggplant, pepper, and tomatoes: Contain plant steroids that block estrogen promotion in breast cancer. Tomatoes and red grapefruit: Contain "lycopines," active chemical ingredients that protect against cancer. Green tea, berries: Contain Catechins that protect against cancer.

HEALTH ISSUE	REMEDIES	
	Vitamins/ Minerals	Spices/Herbs/ Kitchen Aids
Candida albicans (irritable bowel syndrome)		Borage and thyme Rosemary: Thought to encourage the immune system. Savory: antibacterial, antifungal, and antiviral.
Canker sores	B_6, niacin, B_2	Sage: Use sage tea for mouth sores (or sore eyes). Or apply one inch of powdered sage against the sore. Apply goldenseal or raw onion to sore.
Capillary fragility		Lemons: Cut 3 lemons into small pieces; add the peelings of 3 more lemons cut small. Boil in 1½ quarts of water for 20 minutes. Steep for 25 minutes; strain and drink 1 cup twice daily for 2 weeks.
Carbuncles	A, B-complex, C, E	
Carpal tunnel syndrome	B_{12}, B_6, calcium, magnesium, zinc	
Cataracts	A, B_2, B-complex, C, E, trace minerals from angelica root	Combine equal parts yellow onion juice with honey. Mix well; use 1 or 2 drops in eyes twice daily. Coconut: Take the fresh juice from a coconut and with an eye dropper apply

HEALTH ISSUE REMEDIES

	Vitamins/ Minerals	Spices/Herbs/ Kitchen Aids
Cataracts (cont.)		as much as the eye can hold, then apply hot wet cloths over the eye. Remain lying down and keep the towels hot for 10 minutes.
		Horseradish: Good for cataracts and inflammation of the eyes. Grate the root and eat raw or make broth.
		Natural cheddar cheese, sage honey: Eat 2 ozs. of cheddar cheese twice daily, put 1 drop of sage honey in each eye.
		Bean pods: 2 ozs. in 1½ quarts water. Boil for 20 minutes and drink 6 ozs. 3 times daily.
Catarrh		Horseradish: 1 tsp. several times.
Catarrhal deafness		Garlic
Celiac disease	B from rice polishings, folic acid, calcium, magnesium, niacin May be caused by selenium deficiency.	Banana: A godsend with celiac. Children are limited in their food intake, but banana goes well and corrects the altered intestinal functions. Apple: Must be finely grated.
Cellulite		Eggplant: Slice and place in slightly salted water for about 20 minutes or more to remove the bitterness.

HEALTH ISSUE   REMEDIES

	Vitamins/ Minerals	Spices/Herbs/ Kitchen Aids
Cellulite (cont.)		Eggplant skin is extreme- ly helpful. Peel the egg- plant ½-inch thick. Boil the peelings until done. Season with kelp or dulse. An excellent antidote to tumors and cellulite. Sage: Add to bathwater. (May also use sage oil.)
Chapped hands	Calcium fluoride, silicon	
Children (naughty) (see also Lead poisoning)		Cranberry juice with cloves, cinnamon, and honey
Children (toe-walking)		Chickpea
Children (who do not talk)		Fresh strawberries
Chilly, after retiring	Magnesium	
Chlorosis	Sodium	
Cholesterol	C, bioflavonoids, B-complex, E, F, choline, inositol, magnesium, lecithin	Cranberries: 2 tbls. cran- berry sauce once daily or 1 cup of juice a day. Alfalfa sprouts: Use to dissolve cholesterol deposits. Apple: Eat 1 a day. Garlic, onions, leek, and chives inhibit cholesterol synthesis and protect against carcinogens.

HEALTH ISSUE | | REMEDIES

Health Issue	Vitamins/ Minerals	Spices/Herbs/ Kitchen Aids
Cholesterol (cont.)		Cayenne: When taken in capsules may reduce buildup. An herbal combination of okra, mole fern, beth root, rhubarb root, and calamus root.
Chorea	A, B$_1$, B$_6$, magnesium	
Chromium poison		Thyme tea: This is an antidote to chromium poison that settles in the brain.
Circulation	Vitamin E deficiency	Cardiac cocktail: 1 tbl. paprika, 1 tbl. vinegar. Gradually substitute cayenne in place of paprika as soon as you can tolerate it. For serious cases take 1 cup of this in warm water twice daily. Tansy: Aids circulation to the uterus. Fennel, ginger: Circulatory stimulants. Rosemary, lily of the valley (*Convallaria majalis*) (homeopathic), and ginseng help circulation. A combination of hawthorn berries, *Equisetum* concentrate, vitamin C, taurine, arginine, chromium picolinate, and selenium, along with aloe vera gel.

HEALTH ISSUE

REMEDIES

Health Issue	Vitamins/ Minerals	Spices/Herbs/ Kitchen Aids
Clots	C, E, bioflavonoids, rutin, and minerals from white oak bark tea	White oak bark tea
Colds	A, C, iodine, calcium, trace minerals from elder-flower and peppermint	Celery: Increases the appetite, good in curing mucous conditions. Combine: Cloves, cinnamon, sage, and bay leaves; boil in apple juice. Kale: Aids resistance to colds; has natural sulfur and lots of vitamins. Lemon balm, garlic, or cayenne pepper: Deter colds, flu if taken at the onset. White and red onions: Make a soup from raw onions, season with Tamari or other broth and eat. Broccoli: Its natural sulfur strengthens resistance to colds. Thyme: For resistance to colds or prevention of colds, take thyme tea (1 cup a day). Grapefruit: Grate the skin of a grapefruit very fine. Add the juice of ½ grapefruit and fill cup with hot water. Grapefruit contains a substance similar to quinine. Indian remedy: For chest cold, mix turpentine and coconut butter to a paste,

HEALTH ISSUE		REMEDIES
	Vitamins/ Minerals	Spices/Herbs/ Kitchen Aids
Colds (cont.)		rub on hot wool cloth, and apply to chest or back.
Cold sores		Carrots: Take two, finely grated, place between 2 layers of cotton cloth and apply to sores. Change every 2 hours. Brewer's yeast, milk, meat, or soybeans: Sources of lysine, which helps block reproduction of herpes virus. Tea bags: Apply wet, black tea bags to canker sores. An herbal combination of olive leaves and yarrow.
Colic		Fennel: Add 1 tsp. seeds to 1 cup water. Bring to boil, then simmer for about 10 minutes. Strain and give children, only 1 tsp. in water. Gentian: Make tea, and give 1 tsp. in warm cup of water to children. Caraway and anise: Combine and make tea. Yam: Soothing properties help colic. Allspice; cinnamon: Both relieve colic. Dill tea: Diluted. Fenugreek tea: Drink.

HEALTH ISSUE	REMEDIES	
	Vitamins/ Minerals	Spices/Herbs/ Kitchen Aids
Colitis	A, C, B-complex from rice polishing, E, F, magnesium, potassium from bran, trace minerals from white oak bark and goldenseal root Take calcium for a spastic colon.	Comfrey tea, fenugreek tea, wild blackberry or red oak bark tea, creamed papaya, charcoal, bananas relieve colitis. Flaxseed tea: Soak flaxseed in plenty of water overnight, then bring to a boil and simmer for 5 minutes. Drink 3 to 4 times a day. Carrots: Boil until done, then blend or mash them, and eat. Also drink 6 to 7 ozs. of carrot juice twice daily.
Collapse, with burning face	Sodium	
Colon, inflammation and irritation	Calcium: Try extra calcium when the abdomen is distended and bloated. Take B_1 to strengthen.	Irish potato peel and flaxseed meal: Boil a handful of potato peelings in plenty of water. Add 1 tbl. of flaxseed meal to 1 quart of potato peel water and drink 1 cup warm during the day until 1 quart is gone. Do this for 10 to 14 days. Rutabaga is excellent for a weak colon. It is food for the friendly bacteria in the colon and strengthens the membranes of the colon. Boil potatoes with rutabagas, mash them, and eat with butter and salt.

Health Issue	Remedies	
	Vitamins/ Minerals	Spices/Herbs/ Kitchen Aids
Colon, inflammation and irritation (cont.)		Nutmeg: Combine ½ tsp. in hot water for distended abdomen (without nausea). Linden flower tea or 12-herb tincture formula[1]: For abdominal tenderness. Pears, rhubarb: Colon cleansers.
Colon, peristaltic movement impaired	Pantothenic acid	
Complaining, about little things	Calcium	
Complexion, cleared		Cucumber juice with water. Or place slices of cucumber over face where needed.
Complexion, general		Drink 16 ozs. prune juice and 1 gallon apple juice each day for 3 days.
Concentration, loss of	B_{12}, B-complex, glutamic acid, niacin	
Confusion	Niacin, C, B-complex, sodium	Ginger tea: Drink ½ cup twice a day.
Congestion		Foot bath with mustard draws blood out of head. For lungs, a mustard plaster with whole wheat flour; also excellent for kidneys.

[1] The herbs include apple tree bark, calamus root, burdock root, pimpernel root, angelica root, cherry bark, rhubarb root, gentian root, aloes, cascara sagrada bark, nutmeg, and myrrh.

HEALTH ISSUE   REMEDIES

	Vitamins/ Minerals	Spices/Herbs/ Kitchen Aids
Conjunctivitis	B₂	Place raw potatoes on eyes (grated or sliced).
Constipation	B, C, sodium, trace minerals	Figs and prunes: Soak 1 fig and 3 to 5 prunes in warm water overnight. Next morning, drink the juice and eat the fruit. Pears: 2 raw pears at bedtime. No water with them. Flaxseed: Soak 1 tbl. flaxseed with 1 tbl. raisins (currants are best) in 1 cup water. Next morning, eat them before breakfast. Or mix and soak flaxseed with prune juice. Take 1 or 2 tbls. daily. Squash with caraway and cream Raw apple: At bedtime chew an apple very carefully and drink a glass of water with it. Oranges, thyme: Good digestive tonics.
Constriction, of urethra	Potassium	
Corns and calluses	A	
Corns on feet, sensitive		Buttercup White cabbage: Grate cabbage, add hot water so it is comfortable to your feet. Soak them for 10 to 20 minutes.

Health Issue	Remedies	
	Vitamins/ Minerals	Spices/Herbs/ Kitchen Aids
Corns on feet, sensitive (cont.)		Lemon: Soak your feet in warm water for about 15 minutes, then cut a small piece of lemon peel and place the inside of it against the corn, tie it on, and let it stay there all night. Do this for 3 nights, and the corn should lift off. Epsom salts: Add to warm water; soak feet. Massage feet, and never wear tight shoes.
Cough, children (cramping)		Boil bread in milk. Make a poultice over throat.
Cough, dry		Potato peelings: Boil, sweeten with honey. Take 1 tbl. several times a day. Onion: Boil cut onions in apple cider vinegar. Add honey. Take 1 tsp. every hour.
Cough, phlegm		Ginger tea several times: 6 ozs.
Cough syrup		Mix 4 drops eucalyptus oil in 1 cup of honey. Take 1 tsp. as needed. Dates, figs, sage: Combine 1 lb. dates, 1 lb. figs, 1 oz. sage, and 4 quarts distilled water. Boil all ingredients for ½ hour, strain, and boil this syrup down to 1 quart. Take as needed.

| HEALTH ISSUE | REMEDIES | |
	Vitamins/ Minerals	Spices/Herbs/ Kitchen Aids
Cough syrup (cont.)		Onion syrup: Take a yellow onion and make a hole in it. Fill hole with honey or raw sugar. Set it in a saucer and after an hour brown tasty syrup drops out. Excellent for children and adults. Honey: Mix ½ honey and ½ lemon juice.
Cough, whooping		Wild cherry bark: 1 tsp. 3 times daily Sage: Add 1 tbl. to 1 pint water; take 1 tsp. 5 times daily *Drosera rotundifolia*: homeopathic remedy.
Cramps, legs	Calcium lactate, B_1	
Cramps, menstrual	Calcium lactate, B_1	
Cramps, soles and palms		Ginger tea
Crippled hands		Mix 1 part sassafras oil with 3 parts almond oil. Massage this mixture daily into hands.
Crohn's Disease	Eat foods rich in vitamin E.	Protozoa Kit Olive leaves: Counteract both protozoa and viral infections.
Crying, involuntary	Calcium	
Crying, spells	Manganese	

Health Issue	Remedies	
	Vitamins/ Minerals	Spices/Herbs/ Kitchen Aids
Curved spine		Sleeping on an oat straw mattress is thought to heal bones and straighten spine. Homeopathic remedy for T.B. residue.
Cuts		Cloves: Anesthetic properties relieve pain. Apple juice and olive oil: Mix and use as an antiseptic.
Cyst formation	Calcium	Trailing arbutus (*Epigaea repens*): Homeopathic remedy.
Dandruff (see also Hair)	E Lack of vitamin B can result in dandruff.	White beets: Cut beets and boil in water until water is almost gone. Strain and take this water to moisten the scalp for 2 to 3 weeks. Coconut oil: Secure a small amount of pure coconut oil; rub in your hair for a few days and dandruff should disappear. Willow leaves: Boil a handful of leaves. Strain and wash your hair and scalp in it. Put a little concoction aside and dampen the scalp a little every day. (I found this recipe in an old herb book. I was amazed at the result.)

HEALTH ISSUE   REMEDIES

	Vitamins/ Minerals	Spices/Herbs/ Kitchen Aids
Deafness	A, B_{12}, E, F, iodine, niacin	
Debility		Ginger tea
Debility, of limbs		Daisy tea: Drink 2 cups daily. Juniper branches: Boil for 45 minutes and add the fluid to bathwater twice a week.
Deep afflictions		Tomato: Use as poultices in deep-rooted afflictions. When stewed, good for liver. Fresh tomatoes are a vitamin C supplier. Green tomatoes in very small quantities are a gland stimulant. Always remove the core and stem. Make a deep insertion. The stem part is poisonous.
Deodorizer	Zinc	Chlorophyll: Everything that is green has chloro-phyll. Take plenty of green drinks or buy liquid chlorophyll to combat body odor. Eat some parsley after onions or garlic.
Depressed feeling	Niacin, B-complex, B_{12}, C, E	
Depression	Take extra pantothenic acid and vitamin B_6.	Two-thirds of all mental cases are kidney cases.

HEALTH ISSUE	REMEDIES	
	Vitamins/ Minerals	Spices/Herbs/ Kitchen Aids
Depression (cont.)		Drink juice of 1 pome-granate in the morning, 1 persimmon at noon, and 1 wineglass full of grape-fruit juice in the evening; keeps you in good humor. Black snakeroot: Indians chewed this root to calm the nerves and to allevi-ate depression. Lemon balm and Daisy tea: A calming effect. Borage tea: Helpful for grief, anxiety, and depression. Anise and thyme teas Oranges, oats, and rose-mary are helpful. Garlic: Burn the garlic skin slowly on an incense burner to help right away; it's a mild tranquilizer. Clove concentrate: Bruise a handful of cloves, steep in boiling water, then simmer for a few minutes. Do not reduce water too much or it will be too strong. Take 1 tsp. added to 1 cup of hot water. Or try clove tea.
Dermatitis		Oatmeal bath: Home remedy for dermatitis.
Desire to stretch frequently	Calcium	

HEALTH ISSUE	REMEDIES	
	Vitamins/ Minerals	Spices/Herbs/ Kitchen Aids
De-wormer		Figs or pomegranate
Diabetes (see your physician before treating yourself for diabetes.)	B_1, B_2, B_6, B_{12}, niacin, C, E, lecithin, potassium, chromium, inositol, magnesium, zinc, acidophilous	Avocado: Combine avocado with agar-agar (dry), lime juice, and raw rolled oats. Drink plenty of distilled water between meals. Blackberry leaf tea, blueberry leaf tea, or oat straw tea: Boil and drink 4 cups daily. Devil's claw: capsules Dwarf leaf tea: Drink 2 cups a day. Garlic: Helps regulate blood sugar levels; known to be beneficial in adult onset diabetes. Paprika (zinc) will save eyesight in diabetics. Take 2 raw string beans daily. Jerusalem artichoke and parsley leaves are good. Watercress: Make a big salad out of one bunch of watercress for lunch. White figs: Make compresses over throat.
Diaper rash	A, D	Vitamin A and D ointment is the best remedy. Be sure to dry diapers in the sunlight after washing.

HEALTH ISSUE

REMEDIES

	Vitamins/ Minerals	Spices/Herbs/ Kitchen Aids
Diarrhea, chronic	B$_6$, C, F, calcium, magnesium	Apples: Raw and finely grated will stop diarrhea in children. Arrowroot starch: Take 1 tsp. arrowroot. Make a paste with water and stir into 7 ozs. boiling water; add applesauce to taste. Blackberries: As juice or as wine; or drink dried Blackberry root tea. Black tea: Drink 1 or 2 cups without sugar, sipped slowly. Black pepper: Use as a tea for running bowels. Iceberg lettuce has a natural opium that is terribly constipating. Oak bark tea; rice gruel; ripe, raw grated apples; slippery elm; strained carrots; cinnamon; cardamom; rice gruel; nutmeg: All relieve diarrhea.
Difficulty speaking and singing	Sulfur	
Difficulty taking a deep breath	Iron	
Difficulty thinking	Calcium	
Digestion	A, B, C, and E	Alfalfa seed: Improves digestion. Use it as a tea after meals. Add 1 tsp.

HEALTH ISSUE

REMEDIES

	Vitamins/ Minerals	Spices/Herbs/ Kitchen Aids
Digestion (cont.)		alfalfa seed to 1 cup cold water, bring to a boil, then turn the heat off. Let sit for 3 to 5 minutes.
		Flaxseed: It's soothing to an irritated digestive tract. It coats, heals, and nourishes. Take 2 tbls. of flaxseed to 1 quart of water. Simmer for 20 minutes, strain, and drink 1 cup of the warm mixture every 2 hours. For best results alternate with carrot juice: 1 hour carrot juice, the next hour flaxseed tea.
		Sage tea: Aids in protein digestion. Drink 1 cup 2 times daily.
		Basil, celery: Aid in digestion of protein, increase appetite, and are good for mucous.
		Zucchini: Wash zucchini and cut into pieces. Steam or boil with a little water; place on plate and sprinkle with ground almonds. Good for weak digestion.
		Fruit skin: Peel pears, apples, pineapples, peaches, apricots (or whatever you have). Take the peelings and simmer 3 to 5 minutes in plenty of water. Drink 7 ozs. several times a day for digestive problems.

HEALTH ISSUE   REMEDIES

	Vitamins/ Minerals	Spices/Herbs/ Kitchen Aids
Digestion (cont.)		Garlic, nutmeg, cardamom, lettuce, spinach, oranges, ginger, thyme, and papaya are digestive aids.
Digestion, in children		Apple concentrate: Take 2 tsps. of concentrate in water before meals.
Dilated blood vessel, on legs (veins)	Calcium fluoride	
Dirty, oily, yellowish skin pigmentation	Calcium fluoride	
Disc trouble	E, B-complex, C, pantothenic acid, B_{12}, sulfur	
Dislike, of children	Manganese	
Dislike, of moisture	Iodine	
Dislike, of opposite sex	Phosphorus	
Dislike, of work	Phosphorus	
Distention of stomach	Potassium	Bananas area good source of potassium.
Distraction by noise	B-complex from rice bran, E, folic acid, F, iron, sulfur, magnesium	
Diuretics		Cucumber: A good diuretic, containing a hormone needed by the pancreas to produce

HEALTH ISSUE   REMEDIES

	Vitamins/ Minerals	Spices/Herbs/ Kitchen Aids
Diuretics (cont.)		insulin. It is a specific for skin troubles. Seeds: Take equal parts of caraway, fennel, and anise; 1 tsp. each in 1 cup of water. Parsley root tea
Diuretics, for kidney stones		Use cucumber juice or tea from ½ avocado leaf. Or take 3 tsps. of brown cord seed and put in 1 pint of water. Allow to steep, then drink 1 cup daily. This is said also to be good for gallstones.
Diverticulitis	B-complex from rice bran, E, folic acid, F, iron, sulfur, magnesium	Eat no wheat; drink fennel tea to relieve bloatedness.
Dizziness	B_1, B_{12}, C, niacin, calcium, iron	Rinse mouth with 1 tbl. of apple cider vinegar.
Dizziness, with deafness		Take 1 tsp. horseradish every morning.
DNA	Folic acid: repairs and strengthens	
Douche, hygiene		Combine 1 pint apple brandy, 1 tsp. sea salt. Shake. Use 2 tbls. to 1 quart water. Excellent.
Dropsy	Potassium, C, E	Broom tops: Take in capsules or as tea. Potato peelings: Boil peelings and drink 6 ozs. twice daily.

HEALTH ISSUE | REMEDIES

Health Issue	Vitamins/ Minerals	Spices/Herbs/ Kitchen Aids
Dropsy (cont.)		Elder flowers: 2 cups daily. Horseradish in apple juice: Take ½ cup 3 times a day. Combine: ½ gallon apple cider; 1 handful parsley, crushed; 1 handful horseradish, crushed; 1 tbl. juniper berries. Put in cider, let stand 24 hours in a warm place before use. Take ½ glass 3 times a day before meals.
Drug addiction		Epsom salts: Place 3 to 5 pounds of Epsom salts in a tub of hot water; let person soak for 20 minutes. From Denmark: Boil equal parts of carrots, onions, potatoes, celeriac (celery root). Take once a day for 7 days. Add salt and butter.
Drug residue	Chromium and vanadium	Lima beans: Make a healthful dish of lima beans, bell peppers, and sweet potatoes. Eat this once a day for 7 days. Chaparral tea: Two cups a day (or capsules) for heroin deposits. Tobacco leaf tea: Add to bathwater. Oats and celery root (celeriac): Eat to combat morphine habit.

HEALTH ISSUE   REMEDIES

	Vitamins/ Minerals	Spices/Herbs/ Kitchen Aids
Dry, mouth and throat	Potassium	Calamus root: Chew a small piece.
Dry, skin	A, C, E, F	
Dull pain (under both shoulder blades)	Iodine	Kelp, baking soda: Rub on painful area.
Duodenal ulcer		Calamus root: Let sit in cold water overnight. Warm it in the morning (do not boil). Drink ½ cup 4 to 5 times daily. Comfrey root tea: 2 cups daily. 12-herb tincture formula[1]
Ear, burning		Cayenne pepper
Ear, general		Violet root
Ear, gland swollen		Flaxseed (ground): Mix flaxseed with salt, put between layers of cloth and apply.
Ear, humming and roaring in	A, B-complex, B_6, C, and P	Club moss tea Onion juice or cabbage juice: Drop 1 or 2 drops of onion juice into the ear for lost hearing. Watercress, figs, and mustard: Cut, mash, and make a poultice over the ear.

[1] The herbs include apple tree bark, calamus root, burdock root, pimpernel root, angelica root, cherry bark, rhubarb root, gentian root, aloes, cascara sagrada bark, nutmeg, and myrrh.

HEALTH ISSUE | | REMEDIES

Health Issue	Vitamins/ Minerals	Spices/Herbs/ Kitchen Aids
Ear, inner		Horsetail: 1 handful, boil and strain. Add to your bath. Soak for 20 minutes.
Ear, pain		Going from one ear, through the head, to the other ear: Plantain. Shooting pain: Violet leaf tea.
Ear, ringing in		Grapefruit: Try eating a piece if you have pain in the temporal region. Drink chamomile tea. Blue flag (*Iris versicolor*) (homeopathic)
Ear, stinging		Violet leaf tea
Ear, swelling (behind)		Take a cloth, moisten it, sprinkle with freshly ground pepper, and apply.
Earache		Garlic oil: Take ½ lb. of peeled and crushed garlic cloves, put in a jar, and cover with olive oil. Close tightly and shake a few times each day for 3 days, storing in warm place. Strain through a clean cotton cloth; store in a cool place. To use: Drop a little in ear. Leave it for only 10 minutes, then remove with cotton. Moisten cloth with oil, sprinkle with black pepper and apply outside the ear as a compress.

HEALTH ISSUE   REMEDIES

	Vitamins/ Minerals	Spices/Herbs/ Kitchen Aids
Earache (cont.)		Rub sassafras oil around ear, not inside.
Ears, frozen		Apply peppermint oil.
Easily fatigued	Iron	
Eczema	A, B-complex, B_6, B_{12}, C, D, F, calcium, magnesium, niacin	Flaxseed: Contains healing oil that can be used externally or internally. Flax oil is also useful. Oil extracted from seeds of borage is available in capsules and is applied to the skin for eczema and other rashes or dry skin. Strawberry leaf tea
Eczema, babies	B_6	
Eczema, behind the ear		Club moss
Eczema, childhood		Pansy (*Viola tricolor*) tea
Eczema, eruptions/ blisters over joints and fingers		Clove water: Drink 3 cups a day. Evening primrose oil
Eczema, feet and legs	Potassium	
Eczema, scalp		Pansy (*Viola tricolor*) tea
Edema of lower eyelids	B_6, C, potassium	Garden radish: Eat 1 before each meal.
Electromagnetic energies, lack of		Iodine herbs (see chapter 16)

HEALTH ISSUE	REMEDIES	
	Vitamins/ Minerals	Spices/Herbs/ Kitchen Aids
Emotional		St. Ignatius' bean (*Ignatia amara*) (homeopathic)
Emotional sensitivity		Thuja tea (*Thuja occidentalis*) (homeopathic)
Emotional upset		Meadowsweet tea: 1 cup sweetened with honey.
Emphysema	A, B-complex, C, E, folic acid, friendly bacteria, aloe vera juice for trace minerals	An herbal combination of garlic, rosehips, rosemary, echinacea root, and thyme, along with an herbal combination of alfalfa seed, blessed thistle, and goldenseal root.
Endometriosis (tumors all through the uterine wall)	B, C, inositol	Dr. Carlton Fredericks says, "Absolutely no car-bohydrates—not even bananas." Take 1,000 mg. choline and 500 mg. inositol with each meal. Stress B with C, 6 a day$_i$. Douche with alum root for bleeding. In 10 days, pain will leave. Keep up for 6 weeks.
Energy	B_1, B-complex, lecithin, pantothenic acid, iron	Grapes supply a lot of energy. Blackstrap molasses pro-vides minerals and iron. Flaxseed: Let ½ tbl. flax-seed steep in ½ pint hot water; drink twice daily.
Enlarged glands	Iodine, C, B-complex, F, pantothenic acid, lettuce water for trace minerals	

HEALTH ISSUE   REMEDIES

	Vitamins/ Minerals	Spices/Herbs/ Kitchen Aids
Enlarged joints	D, calcium	
Enlarged liver, spleen (without pathological changes)	Calcium fluoride	
Enlarged ovaries	E, manganese	
Enlarged uterus	Calcium fluoride	Yarrow tea
Enteritis	B-complex from rice bran, B_2, friendly bacteria, oak bark tea for trace minerals, niacin	
Environmental poisons (see also Fallout)		Willow leaves Cinnamon removes fall-out. Toast 1 slice of bread very brown, butter it, and sprinkle with cinnamon.
Enzymes		Pineapple: Enzyme supplier.
Epilepsy		Mistletoe (*Viscum album*) (homeopathic)
Epileptic type of convulsive disorder	B_6, calcium, magnesium	
Equilibrium (restore)		Peppermint: Rub on back of neck.
Eustachian tube, catarrh		Rose petals
Eustachian tube, stuffed		Alfalfa seed tea: Several cups. Cayenne pepper.

HEALTH ISSUE	REMEDIES	
	Vitamins/ Minerals	Spices/Herbs/ Kitchen Aids
Excessive thirst	Sodium	
Exhaustion, nervous	B-complex, B_{12}, C, E, F, pantothenic acid	Silicon herbs Whey powder: Take 1 tbl. twice daily. Thyme tea: Drink.
Eyelids, chronic infection	A, B-complex, C, calcium	
Eyelids, glued in morning	A, calcium fluoride	
Eyelids, inflamed		Apply castor oil
Eyelids, swollen		Primrose: Place well-beaten egg whites over closed eyes.
Eyes, aching	Calcium fluoride	
Eyes, atrophy of the optic nerve		Bathe eye in tobacco water.
Eyes, blood and lymph		Carrots: Not in excess. Drink the juice slowly. Also help prevent night blindness.
Eyes, burning	A, B_2, eyebright herb for trace minerals	Eyebright tea: Drink 2 cups daily.
Eyes, cataract (see also Cataracts)		Bean pods: 2 oz. bean pods in 1 ½ quarts water, boil for 20 minutes, and drink 6 oz. 3 times daily.
Eyes, conjunctivitis		Raw potato: Place on eye.
Eyes, and digestion		Bell pepper (increases pepsin)

HEALTH ISSUE	REMEDIES	
	Vitamins/ Minerals	Spices/Herbs/ Kitchen Aids
Eyes, dirty yellow color		Celandine (*Chelidonium majus*) (homeopathic)
Eyes, farsighted		Lack of protein: You need more.
Eyes, fibrillation	B_1	
Eyes, hemorrhage		Linden flower tea: Drink cool, 2 cups daily.
Eyes, inflamed		Castor oil: Apply to eyes. Elder flower tea: Apply externally and drink as well. Eyebright tea Red potato slices: Apply to eye. White lily leaves: Apply to eye.
Eyes, loss of vision from diabetes	Zinc	Paprika (Hungarian is best.)
Eyes, loss of vision from tobacco	B_{12}, folic acid	
Eyes, muscular weakness		Linden flower tea: Drink cool, 2 cups daily.
Eyes, pain		Raw Potato: Poultice over eye.
Eyes, pinkeye		Potatoes: Raw, grated potatoes over the closed eye. You may also take thin slices of raw potato and cover eye. It will release pain and the redness will go away. Red potatoes are best.

Health Issue	Remedies	
	Vitamins/ Minerals	Spices/Herbs/ Kitchen Aids
Eyes, pressure	Manganese	Pokeroot tea: Drink 1 cup twice daily. Red clover tea
Eyes, problems		Cardamom: Eye and brain food. Raw red potatoes: Grate 1 raw potato and use as a poultice over the eyes for 1 hour every day. Will improve eye conditions. Even cataracts have been known to be greatly benefited.
Eyes, retinal bleeding	C, B_1, bioflavonoids, rutin	Raw potato compresses Paprika (Hungarian): 1 tsp. on your food 3 times daily.
Eyes, sensation of gauze over		Linden flower tea: Drink 2 cups daily.
Eyes, strengthener needed		Angelica root tea: Drink ½ cup twice daily. Fennel: Use as an eye-wash. Make a tea, strain, then bathe eyes with it. Improves eyesight. Maple syrup; rosemary Sunflower seeds: Nibble about ½ cup daily. Helpful for eyestrain and sensitivity to light.
Eyes, sties		Eyebright (*Euphrasia officinalis*) (homeopathic) Castor oil Burdock root tea: Drink it and apply it.

HEALTH ISSUE   REMEDIES

	Vitamins/ Minerals	Spices/Herbs/ Kitchen Aids
Eyes, sties (cont.)		Black tea: Make a poultice, place moist over the eye, and bandage it overnight.
Eyes, strain	A, B_2, C, E	Sunflower seed: Nibble about ½ cup daily.
Eyes, tired	A, B_2, C, E, eyebright for trace minerals	Pure maple syrup: Take ½ to 1 tsp. Dr. Hohensee promoted the following formula: Juices of ½ potato, ½ onion, and ½ green pepper. Drink 8 ozs. of this ½ hour before supper. Eyes get clearer after 30 days. Red potatoes: Apply raw poultices.
Eyes, trauma (hard blow)		Comfrey root compresses
Eyes, twitching eyelid	B_6	Elder flower tea
Eyes, watering (excessive)		Euphrasia and eyebright: Homeopathic
Eyes, weak		Rue tea: Drink 2 cups daily.
Facial muscle, pain	B_{12}, folic acid	
Facial neuralgia		Raw plantain juice: Apply over painful area.
Faint (all feeling gone)		Bloodroot tea: Take one cup twice daily.
Fainting	E, B-complex, B_6, manganese	Lavender tea

HEALTH ISSUE | REMEDIES

	Vitamins/ Minerals	Spices/Herbs/ Kitchen Aids
Fallout (see also Environmental poisons)	C (from cloves)	Cinnamon removes fallout. Toast one slice of bread very brown. Butter it and put cinnamon on it. You may also use brown sugar. This counteracts radiation. Cloves: Boil in cranberry juice and willow leaves. Use in bathwater or as tea. Seaweed and miso soup have a neutralizing effect on radiation overdose. Soda, salt: Combine 1 tbl. baking soda and 1 tbl. salt in a tub of warm water. Soak for 15 to 20 minutes. Wash or shower with fresh water. Soda, borax: Combine 3 tbls. baking soda, 1 tbl. borax. Mix and take ½ tsp. before meals.
Fat deposits (see also Antifat)		Carrot juice: Through vitamin and mineral content, it helps the body release energy from the fat stores. It does not store well and should be made up fresh and drunk immediately if possible.
Fatigue, chronic	A, B-complex, B$_{12}$, C, E, pantothenic acid, niacin, folic acid, trace mineral	
Fatty liver	A, B-complex, B$_{12}$, C, E, choline, inositol, lecithin, sulfur (as sulfur baths), trace minerals from buckthorn tea	Buckthorn tea

HEALTH ISSUE   REMEDIES

	Vitamins/ Minerals	Spices/Herbs/ Kitchen Aids
Faultfinding tendency	Iron	
Fear	Niacin, B-complex, C, magnesium	Rosemary tea, cinnamon tea, lavender tea: Equal parts.
Fear, of examination		Cashew nuts: Chew nuts.
Fear, of the unknown	Phosphorus	
Feeling of body and soul being separate		*Thuja occidentalis* (homeopathic)
Feeling of intoxication		Valerian root tea
Feeling too cold		Seaweed or kelp, cayenne (in hot water)
Feeling too hot		Motherwort tea
Feet, aching	Benzene	Hot pepper: If hot peppers upset your stomach, sprinkle hot peppers on the soles of your feet and put on your socks. Hot peppers and radishes contain benzene, which is needed for proper functioning of feet and sinuses.
Feet, burning	Niacin, B-complex, C, magnesium	Tomato: Try tomato slices on the soles of your feet.
Feet, cramps	Sulfur	Put sulfur or cayenne pepper in your socks. Mullein leaf tea
Feet, feeling of deadness		Bathe feet in potato water.

HEALTH ISSUE	REMEDIES	
	Vitamins/ Minerals	Spices/Herbs/ Kitchen Aids
Feet, painful		Lemon juice: Add 3 tsps. of lemon juice (or vinegar or boric acid) to 1 quart of water. Rinse your feet in this solution twice daily. It is supposed to help soothe and refresh sensitive skin. Tomatoes: Apply ripe, mashed, to the soles of feet; or just apply a few slices. Bandage to feet and leave on all night. Soreness should be gone the next morning.
Feet, swollen		Male fern root: Boil 2 ozs. fern in 3 quarts water for 30 minutes. Strain and let cool so it is comfortable to your feet. Bathe feet in it. Save liquid for the next day. Reduces morning swelling. Vinegar: Use vinegar water compresses for feet swollen at night.
Female, bleeding		Okra: Two tbls. cooked okra 3 times a day regulates female bleeding. You can get okra tablets in your health food store. Also good for general female complaints. Orange peeling tea: Used to stop female hemorrhages. See your doctor.

| HEALTH ISSUE | REMEDIES | |
	Vitamins/ Minerals	Spices/Herbs/ Kitchen Aids
Female, trouble (infection) (see also Uterus)		Nettle tea: Known for its antifungal and antiviral properties.
Fever	A, C, bioflavonoids, calcium lactate, trace minerals from raw potatoes	In all fever diseases, there should be a fasting period of two days. Patient needs plenty of liquids, such as: diluted apple juice, diluted grape juice, herb tea with honey, cherry juice, fresh orange juice, lime, and lemonade. Balm (*Melissa officinalis*) tea: 2 cups Coriander, marjoram, and willow bark teas Feverfew tea: 2 cups Garlic: In capsules Gentian: Cools the body and maintains digestive functions. Herbal spice tea: Use equal parts cardamom, cloves, and a little black pepper. Lemon juice: Hot, with honey. Pleurisy root reduces fever.
Fever, blisters	B_2	
Fever, children		Yellow jessamine (*Gelsemium sempervirens*) (homeopathic) *Echinacea angustifolia* (homeopathic)

HEALTH ISSUE	REMEDIES	
	Vitamins/ Minerals	Spices/Herbs/ Kitchen Aids
Fever, and flu	C	Onion: Make an onion soup. This soup will bring vitamin C to work.
Fever, intermittent		Holly tea
Fever, reduced		Pleurisy root
Fever, tick		Chaparral: Take 3 tablets 3 times daily for one month.
Feverish feeling (see also Headache)		Ginger, black pepper, honey
Fibroid tumor		Goldenrod tea Calendula (2 parts), yarrow (1 part), nettle (1 part): Mix and drink 1 quart daily for 4 weeks.
Finger, pain (acute)		St. John's wort (*Hypericum perforatum*)
Finger, swollen		Iodine herbs (see chapter 16)
Fingernails, chewing habit	Calcium	Carrots and cauliflower are calcium-rich foods.
Fingernails, flattened	Iron	
Fingernails, ridged		Silicon herbs (see chapter 16)
Fingernails, split	Sulfur	
Fingernails, thin	Sulfur	
Fingertips, chapped		Buttercup (*Ranunculus bulbosus*) (homeopathic)

HEALTH ISSUE   REMEDIES

	Vitamins/ Minerals	Spices/Herbs/ Kitchen Aids
Fissured tongue	Iron, B-complex	
Fissures, in mouth	B_2	
Flatulence (see also Hysterical flatulence)		Dill, anise, star anise: Equal parts, make tea.
Flatus		Allspice
Flu	Vitamin C for prevention.	Cayenne helps prevent colds/flu. Garlic and onion: Stimulate production of a detoxifying enzyme. Grapefruit: Freshly squeezed grapefruit diluted with water. Equal parts water and grapefruit juice will ease the flu. Lettuce leaves: Take leaf lettuce and boil it in plenty of water. Drink 6 ozs. every hour. Oranges contain vitamin C. Red onion soup: Cut 1 large yellow onion in small pieces; cover with 2 quarts water; simmer for ½ hour. Strain and add honey to taste. Drink 2 cups every 2 hours until flu is gone.
Food, poisoning		Ginger tea with honey: Drink. Vinegar: Take 2 tsps. apple cider vinegar in 1 glass water (no honey) and sip. Repeat every hour until all signs of food poisoning are gone.

HEALTH ISSUE	REMEDIES	
	Vitamins/ Minerals	Spices/Herbs/ Kitchen Aids
Food, poisoning (cont.)		In case of severe vomiting: Moisten cloth with warm vinegar and apply to abdomen. For botulism: Combine 6 parts pokeroot and 3 parts sarsaparilla; make strong tea. Take ½ tbl. every ½ hour.
Forgetfulness		Sage tea: Drink 2 cups a day. Mustard seeds Carbonate of Ammonia (homeopathic)
Freckles		Lemon: Rub stain with a few drops of lemon.
Frightened, easily		Elder flowers: 1 small cup twice daily
Frostbite	K_2 from alfalfa, niacin	Lentils: Use as compress. Calamus root: Soak in calamus root tea.
Fungus		Fungus grows in an alkaline medium. Natural antibiotics are grapefruit, garlic, willow, radish, chlorophyll, and bee pollen. Asparagus: Take 2 tbls. twice daily. Concord grape juice: Drink 3 glasses daily.
Gallbladder		Artichoke: Increases flow of bile.

HEALTH ISSUE   REMEDIES

	Vitamins/ Minerals	Spices/Herbs/ Kitchen Aids
Gallbladder (cont.)		Lemon juice: Fresh lemon juice in 1 cup of hot water taken first thing in the morning will empty your gallbladder and start the day on a happy schedule. Two tsps. of lemon juice before each meal will strengthen the gallbladder. Radishes: Insufficient bile output can be aided by eating one small red radish (or white) before each meal. Pumpkin seeds: Take 1 heaping tsp. ground pumpkin seeds, cover with 7 ozs. of hot water, and drink slowly. Two cups a day are needed. Horseradish: Raw or dried will aid gallbladder.
Gallbladder, chronic trouble, obstructions, or pain		Celandine (*Chelidonium majus*) (homeopathic)
Gallstones		*First day:* 8 A.M. 1 glass (18 oz.) apple juice 10 A.M. 2 glasses (16 oz.) apple juice 12 NOON 2 glasses (16 oz.) apple juice 2 P.M. 2 glasses (16 oz.) apple juice 4 P.M. 2 glasses (16 oz.) apple juice 6 P.M. 2 glasses (16 oz.) apple juice

HEALTH ISSUE   REMEDIES

	Vitamins/ Minerals	Spices/Herbs/ Kitchen Aids
Gallstones (cont.)		(Juice should be natural, without chemicals.)
		Second day: Same procedure as the first day. No food. At bedtime, 4 ozs. olive oil. You may wash the olive oil down with hot lemon juice.
		Black radish, olive oil: Take 2 tbls. grated black radish blended with 1 tbl. olive oil. Take 20 minutes before meals for gallstones.
Gangrene		Echinacea: In capsules.
		Tomatoes: Raw, mashed tomatoes every 2 hours over the gangrene, then 1 hour rest. Leave on all night.
		Tobacco leaves: Poultice of tobacco leaves crushed (heals in 10 days).
		Willow leaves: Apply directly as a compress.
Gas, in stomach and intestines	Sodium, magnesium	
Gas, pain		Allspice relieves gas.
		Certo: Add to ½ glass of apple juice and drink as needed.
		Rue tea: 1 cup with meals. (Do Not Use During Pregnancy.)
Gastric indigestion		Copper herbs (see chapter 16)

HEALTH ISSUE	REMEDIES	
	Vitamins/ Minerals	Spices/Herbs/ Kitchen Aids
Gastric ulcer		Cabbage: Very useful because it contains vitamin U. Cabbage juice: Freshly made cabbage juice, 6 ozs. before meals. Carrots: Nothing to eat but cooked carrots for 7 days. Potato juice: Freshly made potato juice, 7 ozs. between meals. Potato soup made with milk.
Gastric upset		Arrowroot: Take a teaspoonful of arrowroot, make a smooth paste with cold milk or water, stir well, and boil. Add a little lime juice just before taking it.
Gastritis (inflammation of stomach lining)	A, B-complex from rice polishings, E, F, lecithin, trace minerals from flaxseed tea	Flaxseed tea
Gastroduodenal catarrh		Bloodroot tea: ½ cup twice daily.
Germicide		Natural germicides: Cinnamon, or an herbal combination of olive leaves and yarrow
Gingivitis	C, bioflavonoids	
Glands, balancer		Mallow leaf tea: Drink 2 cups daily.

HEALTH ISSUE	REMEDIES	
	Vitamins/ Minerals	Spices/Herbs/ Kitchen Aids
Glands, enlarged	Iodine, C, B-complex, F, pantothenic acid, lettuce water for trace minerals	
Glands, food for		Avocado: Serve without butter or oil. Chicken, chickpeas, sesame seeds, sunflower seeds, sweet potatoes, yams Yucca: Similar to cortisone and is an adrenal gland food.
Glands, stimulant		Barberries: In capsules or as tea. Dandelion root
Glands, swelling in neck		Yellow onion/banana: Bake yellow onion in oven until done. Mash and apply to throat as a poultice, or bake a banana and do the same.
Glands, swollen		Watercress: Juice, 1 tbl. 5 times daily. Salad, eaten with a slice of buttered toast. Marjoram Plantain leaves: Make an oil with these and apply. Plantain neutralizes poisons. Or boil and mix with salt; then use as a compress. Tomato: Place slice on swelling. Fenugreek seeds: Crush and combine with hot milk. Use as a poultice.

HEALTH ISSUE   REMEDIES

	Vitamins/ Minerals	Spices/Herbs/ Kitchen Aids
Glandulars in herbology		Dandelion root: Stimulates glands. Alfalfa seed tea: Nourishes glands. Yucca: Similar to cortisone—adrenal gland food.
Glandular system		Mullein leaf tea: Drink 2 cups daily.
Glandular tissue (strengthener)		Saw Palmetto (*Sabal serrulata*) (homeopathic) or in capsules
Glandular weakness		Sage tea: Drink 1 cup daily.
Glaucoma	A, B-complex, B$_2$, C, bioflavonoids, E	Restrict sweets as your physician tells you to. Yellow onion: Take a thin slice of yellow onion and hold over closed eyes. When tears come, take onion away and wash eyes in fresh, cold water. Do this every day for several weeks. No sugar of any kind if you have glaucoma.
Globulin deficiency	Pantothenic acid	
Gluteal muscle, emaciated		Chickpea (*Lathyrus sativus*) (homeopathic)
Goiter	A, B-complex, calcium, kelp	Agar-agar: 1 tsp. twice daily. Also cool compresses overnight. Pokeroot tea: Drink 2 cups daily.

HEALTH ISSUE	REMEDIES	
	Vitamins/ Minerals	Spices/Herbs/ Kitchen Aids
Gonorrhea		Black walnut tea: 4 cups daily
Good health		Dates and milk
Gout	B-complex, C, E, pantothenic acid, sour cherries for minerals	Onion: Make raw onion poultice over afflicted area. Leave it on all night. Hydrangea root tea: 2 cups daily. Comfrey root tea: 3 times daily.
Gout and stone remedy		Combine 1 quart apple cider, 1 tsp. hydrangea root: Let these stand for 12 hours, bring to a boil, simmer. Take ½ cup 3 times daily. Sour cherries: Take one small dish of sour cherries every morning for 3 weeks.
Graying hair		Sage tea: Drink and rinse through hair. Nettle tea: Drink and rinse through hair.
Grief, apprehension	Magnesium	Borage
Gripping sensation in limbs	Manganese	
Gum disease		Blue vervain (*Verbena hastata*) tea: Make strong and hold a small portion in mouth several times daily. Parsley tea: Use as above. Epsom salts: Hold a weak solution of Epsom salts in your mouth.

HEALTH ISSUE   REMEDIES

	Vitamins/ Minerals	Spices/Herbs/ Kitchen Aids
Gum disease (cont.)		Mulberry: Take 2 oz. twigs and cut into small pieces. Boil in 1 qt. white grape juice for 30 min- utes. Cool, take 1 tbl. every 2 hours. Swish in mouth before swallowing.
Gums, sore		Hyssop tea: Hold in mouth several times daily.
Hair	A, B-complex, F, kelp for trace minerals	
Hair, brittle	A	Nettle tea: Wash hair with it.
Hair, coloring		Nettle leaves
Hair, dandruff (white, scaly)		Nettle; Willow leaf tea
Hair, dull	Sulfur	
Hair, falling out	Sodium	Could be a sign of an underactive thyroid. Eat high protein, no sugar at all, and plenty of yogurt.
Hair, graying	C, E, B-complex, folic acid, B_{12}, PABA, pan- tothenic acid, copper, kelp	Iodine herbs (see chapter 16): To retain natural color.
Hair, loss		Nettle tea Sarsaparilla Wormwood tea: Drink and rinse with cooled tea. Brew 2 tbls. in 1 quart of water for 25 minutes.

HEALTH ISSUE | REMEDIES

Health Issue	Vitamins/ Minerals	Spices/Herbs/ Kitchen Aids
Hair, loss (cont.)		Cool before moistening the scalp. Silicon herbs (see chapter 16) Could be a sign of under-active thyroid. Eat high protein with no sugar at all and plenty of yogurt.
Hair, loss (preventive)		Rosemary: 1 pint of boiling water over 1 ounce of rosemary; mix into solution of 2 tbls. baking soda, strain, and use as a hair rinse to prevent premature baldness. Thyme tea: Prevents or stops hair loss.
Hair, oily	B_2	Wild hops
Hair, tonic		Nettle tea
Halitosis	B-complex, choline, inositol, chlorophyll	Chew juniper berries, caraway seed, or parsley leaves. Rosemary tea: gargle.
Hallucination		Cashew (*Anacardium occidentale*) nuts: Chew nuts thoroughly. Nights: Valerian root.
Hangover		Borage, thyme tea, cucumber: All help relieve a hangover. Fennel tea: Make, strain, and put in bathwater to detoxify the body and release toxic waste.

HEALTH ISSUE   REMEDIES

	Vitamins/ Minerals	Spices/Herbs/ Kitchen Aids
Hay fever	A, B-complex, C, pantothenic acid, sodium	Carrots: Cut 3 carrots and cover with 1 quart water and boil for 20 minutes. Drink this broth as an exchange for the vegetable broth suggested. Vegetable broth: Every half hour drink 4 ozs. of pure water. Do this for 2 days. Then make yourself a vegetable broth and drink on the full hour 6 ozs. of broth and on the half hour 4 ozs. of water. Clover tea, red onion soup, spikenard tea relieve hay fever. Wild plum tree bark: 2 ozs. to 1 quart of water. Boil down to 1 cup, add 1 cup of honey or maple or brown sugar and boil down again. Take 1 tbl. 4 times daily or as needed. Cherry bark tea: 2 cups daily.
Hay fever, with asthma		Damask rose: 2 tbls. 4 times daily.
Hay fever, with profuse, yellow discharge		Fenugreek Nettle tea
Headache		Nerve root (lady's slipper) tea Lavender: Applied hot will relieve almost any local pain. Also drink as a tea. Lavender oil: Applied to temples.

HEALTH ISSUE   REMEDIES

	Vitamins/ Minerals	Spices/Herbs/ Kitchen Aids
Headache (cont.)		Brazilian cocoa (guarana) tea: 1 cup when headache starts. Marjoram reduces headache.
Headache, back of head	Potassium	Might indicate liver or gallbladder trouble.
Headache, dull	Iodine	
Headache, front of head		Might indicate kidney or bladder trouble.
Headache, left side of head		Alfalfa tablets
Headache, middle of head		Indicates intestinal trouble.
Headache, migraine (see Migraine)		
Headache, more frequent in the afternoon	Calcium	
Headache, on one side of head		Allergic reaction to something. Allspice: Crush, take ½ tsp. in juice twice daily.
Headache, radiating from one point		Black tea: 1 cup Vinegar: Wet a handkerchief with half vinegar and half water.
Headache, right side of head		Celandine (*Chelidonium majus*) tea: 1 cup daily. Orange: Peel and eat ½ at a time.

HEALTH ISSUE   REMEDIES

	Vitamins/ Minerals	Spices/Herbs/ Kitchen Aids
Headache, top of head		Indicates intestinal trouble.
Headache, with nausea		Blue flag (*Iris versicolor*) (homeopathic)
Hearing, dull	Iron	
Hearing, loss (hard of hearing)	Manganese (preventive), zinc	Beth root tea: 2 cups daily. Horseradish: 2 drops of fresh horseradish juice in each ear. Try calendula or marigold.
Hearing, rheumatic deafness		Garlic oil: Drench some cotton with garlic oil and put into ear. Wood betony: 2 cups daily. Mistletoe (*Viscum album*) (homeopathic)
Hearing, ringing in ear		Blue flag (*Iris versicolor*) (homeopathic)
Hearing, shrill (high-pitched)		Violet leaf tea: 2 cups daily.
Heart, attack		Compresses to the heart with vinegar water until physician arrives.
Heart, broken		Poplar (balm of Gilead) buds: Carried in pocket or as tea.
Heart, chest pressure	Iodine	
Heart, cramp	Calcium	Fennel: Fennel seed or anise as tea.

HEALTH ISSUE · REMEDIES

Health Issue	Vitamins/ Minerals	Spices/Herbs/ Kitchen Aids
Heart, enlarged	B_1	Asparagus: Take 2 tbls. 2 times daily.
Heart, extra beats or too fast	B_1	
Heart, fibrillation		Rosemary tea Chew on basil herb or cinnamon sticks. Lemon juice with cloves. Coal water: Put on face.
Heart, food		Hawthorn berries, chickweed, motherwort, capsicum, cramp bark (herbal formula)
Heart, general health	E, B-complex, C, magnesium, calcium, lecithin	Olives: Rich in potassium.
Heart, irregularity (See your physician.)	Biotin	Chew basil or cinnamon pieces. Rosemary tea; lemon water with cloves. Basil tea or in capsules
Heart, muscle		Hawthorn berry tea: 2 or 3 cups daily Rosemary tea: 2 cups daily
Heart, nervous palpitation	B-complex, B_6, lecithin, magnesium, calcium, and trace minerals from valerian root	Rue tea (Not during pregnancy)
Heart, pain (irregularity)		Chew basil or cinnamon pieces; rosemary tea; lemon water with cloves. See your physician.

Health Issue	Remedies	
	Vitamins/ Minerals	Spices/Herbs/ Kitchen Aids
Heart, palpitations		Cloves: Boil cloves in fresh or frozen lemon juice. Take 1 tsp. in 4 ozs. of water several times daily.
Heart, strengthener		Cowslip (2 parts), lavender (1 part): Make tea using 1 tsp. per cup and drink 2 to 3 cups daily.
Heart, tonic		To restore electrical part of heart: 4 tbls. cane sugar, 4 tbls. beet sugar, 4 tbls. corn sugar, 2 tsps. kosher or sea salt, and 2 tsps. baking soda. Take 1 tsp. 2 to 3 times daily.
Heart, valves		Blue malva tea: Drink 1 cup twice daily for 6 weeks.
Heart, weakness (slow pulse)		Take 1 quart of water, add 2 tbls. vinegar. Wet a small towel and apply over chest close to the heart. Cover with woolen cloth. Change every hour. Results after several hours.
Heart, weakness or aches (or when overworked)		Parsley wine: Ten long-stemmed parsley, cut into ½-inch pieces (leaves and stems are used), cover with 1 quart natural white wine. Add 1 tbl. apple cider vinegar and bring to a boil. Simmer for 10 minutes, then add ¾ cup of honey. Boil again for 5 more minutes. Strain wine and pour into hot sterile

HEALTH ISSUE   REMEDIES

	Vitamins/ Minerals	Spices/Herbs/ Kitchen Aids
Heart, weakness or aches (cont.)		bottles. Close tightly or set in refrigerator. (Caution: Wine will run over easily while heating; stay with it.) Take 3 tbls. 2 to 3 times daily.
Heartburn		Ginger: Take right after eating. Start with a small amount and work up to the right dosage for you. Slippery elm tea Potato: Eat a slice of raw potato when you have heartburn.
Heaviness, eyelids		Violet leaves
Heaviness, stomach		Ginger tea
Heels, aching		Pokeroot tea: ½ cup twice daily
Heels, pain		Club moss tea: 1 cup daily When sitting: Valerian tea—1 cup daily. Achilles tendon: St. Ignatius' bean (*Ignatia amara*) (homeopathic)
Hemorrhage, bladder	Magnesium	Peach tree bark tea: 3 cups daily. Comfrey root tea: 3 cups daily.
Hemorrhoids	B_6, calcium, chlorophyll	Almonds: Eat 3 a day to prevent and eliminate hemorrhoids.

HEALTH ISSUE

REMEDIES

	Vitamins/ Minerals	Spices/Herbs/ Kitchen Aids
Hemorrhoids (cont.)		Stone root (*Collinsonia canadensis*) tea, or in capsules. Dandelion root tea: Brew 15 minutes and drink 2 cups daily. Garlic: Oil a clove and insert it into the rectum each night for several nights in a row. Ginger tea: Relieves hot and painful hemorrhoids. Cranberries: Make a poultice; place over external hemorrhoids. Sage: Make a pillow, fill with sage leaves, and keep it in place overnight. Potato: Slice and dip in oil to lubricate and insert into rectum.
Hepatitis, infectious		Calendula (marigold) tea: With fresh lemon juice and distilled water. Add honey to taste. Drink 1 quart or more daily for 1 week. No fried foods or alcohol and keep warm.
Hernia		Mistletoe, horsetail: Combine and apply as poultice overnight.
Heroin, deposits		Chaparral tea: 2 cups daily or in capsules. Tobacco leaf tea: Add to bathwater.

HEALTH ISSUE	REMEDIES	
	Vitamins/ Minerals	Spices/Herbs/ Kitchen Aids
Herpes, general	C, E, zinc, lysine (500 mg. once a day)	Buck bean tea: 1 cup daily. Club moss; Buttercup (*Ranunculus bulbosus*) (homeopathic) An herbal combination of olive leaves and yarrow.
Herpes, labialis (with itching/sensation of heat)		Nettle tea
Herpes II, blister type		Buttercup (*Ranunculus bulbosus*) (homeopathic) Black walnut tea
Herpes Zoster (see also Shingles)	B-complex, chlorophyll, B_1, magnesium, calcium	Houseleek: In soup or salad. Blue flag (*Iris versicolor*) (homeopathic)
Hiccups		Blow into a paper bag. Vinegar: A few drops on 1 tsp. of sugar. One spoonful in some water. Anise: Make 1 cup of anise tea and sip slowly. Orange: Cut in half; squeeze juice from ½ orange into a glass and drink slowly. Repeat with other half if necessary. Pineapple juice relieves hiccups.
High blood pressure (due to kidney) (see also Blood Pressure, high)		Club moss tea

HEALTH ISSUE   REMEDIES

	Vitamins/ Minerals	Spices/Herbs/ Kitchen Aids
Hip, pain (to feet)		Cayenne pepper: Put in socks.
Hives (see Urticaria)		
Hoarseness (see also Laryngitis; Voice, hoarse)		Drink ginger tea with honey. Plantain tea: Make it strong and sip. It neutralizes poison. Black bean juice: Take black beans and boil them in plenty of water (1 pound of beans to 1 gallon of water); boil for 1 hour, strain. Drink the juice, 6 ozs., 3 to 4 times daily. Eat beans in another dish or in soup. Glycerin: 1 tbl. in hot water; gargle often.
Homesickness		Cayenne pepper: Add to food or sprinkle in shoes.
Hookworm		Thyme tea: Two cups strong tea followed by a dose of Epsom salts. Take Epsom salts ½ hour after the tea.
Hormones, female		Black cohosh, rice polishings Booster: ½ cup ground cashews, 2 tbls. rice polishings, 2 cups water or apple juice. Blend in blender, add honey if wanted. Gives women charm and femininity.

HEALTH ISSUE	REMEDIES	
	Vitamins/ Minerals	Spices/Herbs/ Kitchen Aids
Hormones, female (cont.)		Supply: pumpkin seeds.
Hormones, male		Sarsaparilla, brewer's yeast Booster: 2 tbls. brewer's yeast; 1 tsp. chia seed, 1 cup cashews, 2 cups tomato juice. Blend in blender. Gives men will power and determination. Supply: pumpkin seeds.
Human papilloma virus (HPV)		An herbal combination of blue flag, blue malva, blue vervain, papaya leaves, and mullein, along with a specific homeo-pathic remedy for HPV. Drink concord grape juice every day. Douche with concord grape juice as well.
Hunger, with nausea		Valerian root tea as needed.
Hungry, but feeling full after a few bites	Choline	
Hydrocephalus		Hellebore tea: Take 1 tsp. 4 times daily.
Hyperactive, children		Thyme tea: 2 cups daily, 1 tsp. to 1 cup. A specific homeopathic remedy for chemical toxins.
Hyper insulinism	A, B-complex, C, pantothenic acid, zinc, sulfur from hops tea	

HEALTH ISSUE	REMEDIES	
	Vitamins/ Minerals	Spices/Herbs/ Kitchen Aids
Hypertension		Onions: Contain a substance called prostaglandin. This is normally produced in the human body and is known to have an anti-hypertensive effect.
Hypochondria		Vanilla: Take 1 vanilla bean, cut in pieces. Boil it in 1 cup of water for 5 minutes. Sweeten with honey. Cherries: Eat morning and night for hypochondria.
Hypoglycemia		Three drops sassafras oil in 1 tbl. fruit juice, twice daily for 4 weeks. Red beets help people with low blood sugar.
Hysteria	Sodium	Passion flowers: 1 cup twice daily. Wood betony
Hysteria, connected with female trouble		Motherwort tea: Drink 1 cup twice daily.
Hysterical flatulence		Valerian root tea, or in capsules
Hysterical spasms, stomach		Valerian root tea, or in capsules
Immune system		Take flaxseed and walnuts to stimulate the immune system. They contain alpha linoleic acid.

HEALTH ISSUE · REMEDIES

	Vitamins/ Minerals	Spices/Herbs/ Kitchen Aids
Impetigo (pus-filled pimples, especially over face and scalp)	A, E, folic acid	Pansy tea and/or as a rinse.
Impotence		Fenugreek seed tablets
Inability to digest sugar	B_2, potassium	
Indifference to life		Pokeroot: Take 1 cup daily.
Indigestion	Sodium	Summer savory Citrus family: To 1 quart water add the juice of 1 grapefruit, 1 lemon, 3 oranges, 2 tbls. milk sugar, 1 cup aloe vera. Drink in small sips; 1 quart per day. Whey: 1 tbl. of whey in a little water helps digestion. Slippery elm tea (for chronic indigestion)
Infant colic (see also Colic)		Caraway and anise seed tea
Infection	Take plenty of pantothenic acid when fighting an infection.	Parsley, black radish, savory, basil: Used to treat infections. Cranberries: Boil and use juice to fight infections. Grapefruit: finely grated skin of 1 grapefruit. Take 1 tsp. and add juice of ½ a grapefruit. Drink 3 times daily to fight infection.
Infection, female trouble		Nettle tea has antifungal, antiviral properties.

HEALTH ISSUE | REMEDIES

	Vitamins/ Minerals	Spices/Herbs/ Kitchen Aids
Infection, low-grade	Sulfur, potassium	Natural antibiotics: Garlic, grapefruit, chlorophyll, parsley and radish, willow, bee pollen extract. Cranberries: Boil and use the juice. Potato: Suck raw potatoes and spit out the pulp. Or make 1 cup raw potato juice, add to 3 cups water, and drink.
Infection, skin		White pond lily: Apply to skin.
Infection, tendency to	A, C, E, bioflavonoids, calcium lactate, minerals from fresh lemon juice	Fresh lemon juice.
Infection, virus		Calendula tea, an herbal combination of olive leaves and yarrow.
Infectious disease, general (see also Prevention, infectious diseases)		Warm milk compresses all over the body. Wrap patient in first layer of warm milk sheet; second layer, woolen blanket; third layer, warm cover. Repeat in 2 hours if needed.
Infectious disease, hepatitis		Calendula (marigold) Fresh lime juice
Infectious disease, lung		Onions: Boil, mash, and place them between 2 layers of cloth. Apply to chest for about 2 hours.

HEALTH ISSUE   REMEDIES

	Vitamins/ Minerals	Spices/Herbs/ Kitchen Aids
Infectious disease, sinus		Pepper and honey: Take 1 tsp. honey and sprinkle with freshly ground pepper. Also good for sniffles.
Infectious disease, staph		Grapefruit: Grate the skin of a grapefruit with a fine grater. Take 1 tsp. and add the juice of ½ grapefruit. Drink this 3 times a day.
Inflammation		Flaxseed, soy products, purslane, and walnuts all reduce inflammation. Fenugreek: Add crushed seeds to hot milk and make poultice. Inflammation of body may point to protozoan infection. Take specific homeopathic remedies for protozoa to help relieve inflammation.
Inflammation, colon		Irish potato peel and flaxseed meal: Make tea.
Inflammation, eye and eyelid		Elder flower (externally). Also, drink 2 cups a day. Use raw potato poultice over eye.
Inflammation, lips and mouth	B_6, niacin	
Inflammation, muscles	C, E, pantothenic acid	
Inflamed nerves		Peppermint tea, peppermint lotion
Inflated intestines	Magnesium	

HEALTH ISSUE	REMEDIES	
	Vitamins/ Minerals	Spices/Herbs/ Kitchen Aids
Influenza	A, C, B-complex, pantothenic acid, minerals from linden blossom tea and mint tea	Linden blossom and mint teas
Injuries, bone, tendon, and muscle		Apply comfrey root compresses.
Injuries, deeper tissue		Daisy tea: Drink 2 to 3 cups daily.
Injuries, nerves		Daisy tea: Drink 2 to 3 cups daily.
Injuries, sinew, tendon, and joint		Apply comfrey root compresses. Arnica is best.
Inner ear		Horsetail bath Apply sassafras oil around ear, not inside.
Insect bites (see also Mosquito bite)		Sage tea: Rub it on. Plantain leaf; Yellow onion Apple: Place a piece of raw apple on the bite. Bee sting: On tongue, 1 tsp. salt. Has prevented many from suffocating. (see also Bee sting) Thyme tea: Use as skin antiseptic. Vinegar: Mix vinegar with flax and apply.
Insect repellent		Parsley tea: Rub on skin.

Health Issue	Remedies	
	Vitamins/ Minerals	Spices/Herbs/ Kitchen Aids
Insomnia	B$_6$, D, calcium lactate, minerals from catnip or valerian root	Squaw vine tea Raspberry tea Eucalyptus oil: 10 drops at bedtime in capsules (for gas). Oats: Boil whole grain oats in plenty of water. Strain the oats and season the water with lemon juice and honey. Oats should have the husks on because the healing part is found in the hull and husks. Oranges: Eating them calms the nerves; useful for insomnia. Thyme, dill, and lemon balm are used for insomnia. Milk: Warm and add 1 tsp. honey; drink before bed.
Insomnia, due to worry		Prickly ash leaf tea: Drink 1 cup at bedtime.
Insomnia, elderly		Passion flower tea: Drink 1 cup at bedtime.
Insomnia, infant		Passion flower tea: Drink 1 tsp. of tea to 1 cup of water.
Insulin producer		Cucumber: Contains a hormone needed to produce insulin.
Intestinal catarrh		Ginger tea

HEALTH ISSUE	REMEDIES	
	Vitamins/ Minerals	Spices/Herbs/ Kitchen Aids
Intestinal difficulties		Potato drink: Boil 2 medium potatoes, cut in pieces, in 1 quart of water, with peelings; pour 4 cups of potato water over 3 tbls. flaxseed (ground) and 6 tbls. bran. Let stand overnight with lemon or orange juice and a small, finely chopped onion. Tastes good and is more nutritious.
Intestinal disorder		Combine 1 cup aloe vera juice, 1 quart water, juice of 1 grapefruit, 3 oranges, 1 lemon, 3 tbls. milk sugar, and honey to taste.
Intestinal mucous		Garlic
Intestines, gripping		Coriander: Chew 5 seeds or brew as a tea.
Intoxication (see also Alcohol)		Honey removes alcohol from the blood extra fast.
Iodine supplier		Fish
Itching, intense		Banana peeling: Rub the inside of the peeling on affected area. Buttercup (*Ranunculus bulbosus*) (homeopathic)
Itching, intolerable		Pansy tea: Drink 1 to 3 cups daily.
Itchy, skin	Potassium	Marjoram

Health Issue | Remedies

	Vitamins/ Minerals	Spices/Herbs/ Kitchen Aids
Jaundice (see also Liver, swollen) See your physician.		Lime: Make fresh lime water. Sweeten with honey. This is all you can drink. Drink 6 to 8 ozs. every hour. Stick with juice until you are extremely hungry. This might take 2 to 3 days. Break the juice diet with a small dish of cooked beets and/or cooked carrots. If you tolerate this, 4 hours later, try a piece of baked potato without butter or sour cream. Continue drinking the lime water. Next day, add a little fat-free yogurt or cottage cheese and some well-done rice. In 1 week, you should be back on your feet. Cucumber juice: Drink 4 or 5 cups to purify the lymphatic system. Artichokes and/or anise oil are good for jaundice. Fringe tree (*Chionanthus virginica*) (homeopathic)
Jaundice, children		Hops tea Chamomile tea
Jaundice, repeated condition	Phosphorus	
Jerking, constant	B_6	Valerian root in capsules Emu oil: Counteracts poisons in central nervous system, including nickel, lead, arsenic, cadmium, mercury, msg, dioxin,

Health Issue	Remedies	
	Vitamins/ Minerals	Spices/Herbs/ Kitchen Aids
Jerking, constant (cont.)		aluminum, uranium, and nitrates. Take 10 drops twice a day.
Joints, lubricant		Combine: 1 tsp. turmeric, 2 tsp. almond oil, 2 tbls. soy milk powder, 1 cup water, salt and honey to taste. Heat this and serve as a hot drink.
Joints, pain	Sulfur	Comfrey root tea: Apply and drink. Comfrey root tincture: Apply. Combine avocado seeds (chopped) and horsetail grass (3 oz.). Boil together in 1 quart of water, down to 1 pint. Add rubbing alcohol and use as a liniment. Simmer laurel beans in any oil and apply over aching joints.
Joints, stiff	Use manganese for joint cracking.	Cabbage: Raw poultice. Grate 2 cups very fine, wrap in cheesecloth, and apply overnight. For best results, do it several nights in a row. Cucumber: The natural sodium makes joints limber. An herbal combination of olive leaves and yarrow.
Joints, swollen		Extract potato juice and boil down to ⅕ original amount. Add glycerin to preserve it. Make a poultice and apply.

Health Issue	Remedies	
	Vitamins/ Minerals	Spices/Herbs/ Kitchen Aids
Joyless appearance	Sulfur	
Kidneys	A, B-complex, C, magnesium, trace minerals from herb teas	Herb teas: Watermelon seed, couchgrass, cornsilk, uva ursi Cranberry juice: Drink plenty every day. Cinnamon warms the kidneys. Cold pressed oils are needed to assimilate the proteins from vegetables. They are food to the kidney.
Kidneys, and/or bladder stones	A, B-complex, stone root tea for minerals (for kidney stones)	Anise: Put 1 tbl. in 1 quart grape juice and simmer for ½ hour. Drink 7 oz. 3 times daily. Parsley tea: Drink for 3 days with no other food. Asparagus: dissolves oxalic acid crystals when they are lodged in the kidneys. Grape juice (dark): 1 cup or 7 ozs., add ½ tsp. cream of tartar. Take 2 ozs. 3 times daily before meals. Dandelion root: Boil 2 tbls. in 1 quart apple juice for 10 minutes. Strain and drink 6 ozs. 3 times daily (for kidney stones). Beets: Boil 5 whole, medium-sized beets in 3 quarts of water for 1 hour. Drink 7 ozs. of the water 3 times daily. Use cucumber juice or tea from ½ avocado leaf. Or

HEALTH ISSUE	REMEDIES	
	Vitamins/ Minerals	Spices/Herbs/ Kitchen Aids
Kidneys, and/or bladder stones (cont.)		take brown corn water—allow to steep, then drink 1 cup daily (diuretic for kidney stones). Chamomile and knotgrass (for kidney stones)
Kidneys, and/or bladder trouble		Celery tops: Eat after each meal for 5 weeks.
Kidneys, bleeding	Choline: Is a methyl donor and increases the metabolism in general, and liver and kidney in particular.	Watermelon seed tea.
Kidneys, catarrhal (inflammation)		Juniper berries Watermelon and seeds: For 2 days, eat nothing but watermelon. Always eat the melon by itself. Indian remedy: One radish 3 times a day.
Kidneys, congestion		Blue vervain (*Verbena hastata*) tea
Kidneys, dysfunction		Asparagus: Boil in plenty of water (2 quarts water to 4 ozs. asparagus) and use the concoction, 1 cup, 4 times daily. Strongly diuretic in action. Horseradish boiled in apple juice gives copious urine if kidney is blocked.
Kidneys, gravel		Blue vervain (*Verbena hastata*) tea Broom tops tea

HEALTH ISSUE REMEDIES

	Vitamins/ Minerals	Spices/Herbs/ Kitchen Aids
Kidneys, impaired function	Potassium, magnesium	
Kidneys, infection		Watermelon: Eat all you want for 2 days; no other food.
Kidneys, trouble		Cranberry juice: Combine ½ cranberry juice, ½ water. Take 7 oz. 3 times daily.
Knees, knocking against each other		Chickpeas (*Lathyrus sativus*) (homeopathic)
Knees, swollen		Cabbage: Grate 2 cups (very fine) and place in cheesecloth. Apply over swollen knee several nights in a row.
Labor, pain	B_1, calcium lactate	
Labor, prolonged	B_1	
Labrynthitis (inner ear) (see also Inner ear)	C, bioflavonoids, B-complex, B_{12}, folic acid, E	
Lack of electromagnetic energies		Iodine herbs (see chapter 16)
Lack of pepsin		Hops tea: Before meals.
Lack of sulfur		Fennel seed: Chew or make tea.
Lactation		Anise can enhance milk production and relieve bloated conditions in nursing child.

HEALTH ISSUE   REMEDIES

	Vitamins/ Minerals	Spices/Herbs/ Kitchen Aids
Lactation (cont.)		Caraway seeds increase mother's milk. Add 1 tsp. seeds to 8 oz. cold water. Bring to boil and simmer for a few minutes. Drink several cups a day. Dill tea: Increases mother's milk. Fennel tea: Promotes lactation and relieves colic in nursing child. Lentils and borage are good for lactation.
Lactation, increase in milk		Blessed thistle tea
Lactation, increase in quality		Alfalfa tea
Laryngitis (see also Hoarseness; Voice, hoarse)		Arnica tincture: 3 to 4 drops in 1 tbl. warm water several times daily. Violet leaf tea: Drink or gargle. Black beans: Juice is good for hoarseness and laryngitis. Red onions relieve laryngitis.
Laryngitis, chronic		*Thuja occidentalis* (homeopathic)
Larynx, tickling		Red onion: Raw or as soup
Laxative		Prunes, apricots: Mix 3 prunes and 3 apricots. Soak overnight and take

Health Issue	Remedies	
	Vitamins/ Minerals	Spices/Herbs/ Kitchen Aids
Laxative (cont.)		this much twice daily. This combination is special.
Lead poisoning		Boil cloves in 1 quart of cranberry juice for 20 minutes. Strain and add 2 tsps. ground cinnamon. Add 1 tsp. cream of tartar, stir. Drink 5 oz. 3 times daily for 12 to 15 days. Then, drink it once a week. For children, 3 oz. 3 times daily. Cabbage: Counteracts lead poisoning. Cranberries are also helpful. (see also Children, naughty) Ivy tea: Ground, 2 cups daily. Homeopathic: *Plumbum metallicum*. An herbal combination of pumpkin seed, okra, rhubarb root, capsicum, peppermint, and dulse.
Legs, blue if hanging down		Chickpeas (*Lathyrus sativus*) (homeopathic)
Legs, cramps	Calcium (for cramps at night); calcium when left leg hurts; magnesium when right leg hurts. Potassium	Club moss (*Lycopodium clavatum*): Wrap as a compress, put in a pillow, or use in homeopathic form. Cramp bark tea Male fern: Foot baths. Eat more fruit. Homeopathic: *Arsenicum album*
Legs, swollen		Lady's mantle

| HEALTH ISSUE | REMEDIES | |
	Vitamins/ Minerals	Spices/Herbs/ Kitchen Aids
Leukemia	Shortage of zinc: Chlorophyll from watermelon rind and seeds	Sulfur herbs (see chapter 16) Okra: Gives strength. Red beets: Valuable factors contribute substantially to the health of the body. Watermelon rind and seeds In all cases, the tailbone should be checked and realigned.
Leukopenia (diminishing of white blood corpuscles)	B_6	
Lice		Mineral oil: Warm; pour over entire scalp. After 10 minutes, shampoo. Then use a fine-toothed comb to gather the suffocated lice. Repeat procedure every 2 days for 10 days. Thyme tea: Use as a skin antiseptic.
Light, cannot bear		*Nux vomica* (homeopathic)
Limbs, paralytic with pain		Skullcap tea: Drink several cups daily. Or take in capsule form.
Listlessness	Calcium	
Liver	A, C, E, potassium, choline, inositol	Apricots, pineapple juice: Use to detoxify liver and pancreas. Soak 1 pound dried apricots in pineapple juice. Next morning, blend mixture. Take this 2 days in a row.

HEALTH ISSUE	REMEDIES	
	Vitamins/ Minerals	Spices/Herbs/ Kitchen Aids
Liver (cont.)		Casaba melon: Take by itself. Carrot juice: Take 6 oz. with 2 tbls. cream, 1 hour after breakfast. Combine: ½ quart carrot juice, ½ quart goat's milk, 1 tbl. molasses per quart. Also, white beans, artichokes, allspice, and apples are helpful.
Liver, ailment		Breakfast: 2 tbls. ground flaxseed, 2 tbls. whey, 2 peeled and finely grated apples. Mix and serve with honey. Healing to the liver and intestines.
Liver, cirrhosis	Selenium	Apply club moss compresses.
Liver, cleanser		Chaparral tea; or capsules
Liver, congestion		Blue vervain (*Verbena hastata*) tea: 2 cups daily.
Liver, constipation due to		Barberry tea: 1 cup with meals.
Liver, cutting pain		Blue flag (*Iris versicolor*) (homeopathic is best)
Liver, damage		Dandelion leaves and stems (not the flowers)
Liver, enlarged		Dandelion as tea or in fresh salads Flaxseed: Place in a little bag, hang it in boiling hot water for 10 minutes.

HEALTH ISSUE   REMEDIES

	Vitamins/ Minerals	Spices/Herbs/ Kitchen Aids
Liver, enlarged (cont.)		Squeeze excess water out and apply over liver area. Cover with a towel.
Liver, enlarged with lots of wind		Senna Chamomile
Liver, food		Dandelion leaves; butternut; stewed tomatoes Celandine (*Chelidonium majus*) (homeopathic)
Liver, hardening of		Cloves: Beneficial when swollen, hard, damaged, or containing tumors. Yams Yucca tablets: For pain in right side.
Liver/pancreas		Nutmeg: Add ½ tsp. to 1 cup hot water; acts as a stimulant. Apricots detoxify liver/ pancreas.
Liver, strengthener		Dandelion root tea
Liver, swollen		Potato: Cook red potatoes, mash them, place between two layers of cloth, and apply warm to the liver. Goldenrod, goldenseal root, cloves (herbal formula) Lime juice: Fresh squeezed from 2 limes, combined with distilled water (1 quart), and

HEALTH ISSUE   REMEDIES

	Vitamins/ Minerals	Spices/Herbs/ Kitchen Aids
Liver, swollen (cont.)		honey to taste. Drink 1 quart or more daily for 7 days. Do not chill. Drink at room temperature. Do not eat any fried foods or alcoholic beverages and keep your feet warm.
Loose teeth	C, bioflavonoids	
Loss of alkali reserves	B_1	Apple cider vinegar: 2 tsps. in 1 cup of water with honey.
Loss of appetite	B_6, B_{12}	
Loss of appetite for meat dishes	Choline	
Loss of breath, under slightest exercise	B_1	
Loss of concentration	B_{12}, folic acid, gotu kola	
Loss of courage	C, calcium	
Loss of energy	B-complex, B_1, lecithin, pantothenic acid	
Loss of eyesight, from diabetes	Zinc	Paprika (Hungarian is best.)
Loss of eyesight, from tobacco	B_{12}, folic acid	
Loss of hearing	A	
Loss of ligament reflexes	B-complex, B, E	

HEALTH ISSUE   REMEDIES

	Vitamins/ Minerals	Spices/Herbs/ Kitchen Aids
Loss of mental energies	B_{12}	
Loss of muscle tone	Phosphorus	
Loss of self-confidence		Club moss
Loss of self-esteem		12-herb tincture formula[1]
Loss of sense of smell	A, sodium	
Loss of stomach acidity	B_1, B-complex, niacin	
Loss of strength in muscles, of arms and legs	B_1	
Loss of taste	A	
Loss of tear secretion	B-complex, kelp for trace minerals	
Loss of temper, over nothing	Sodium	
Loss of temperature	B-complex, kelp for trace minerals	
Loss of willpower	Calcium	
Low blood pressure (see Blood Pressure, low)		

[1] The herbs include apple tree bark, calamus root, burdock root, pimpernel root, angelica root, cherry bark, rhubarb root, gentian root, aloes, cascara sagrada bark, nutmeg, and myrrh.

HEALTH ISSUE   REMEDIES

	Vitamins/ Minerals	Spices/Herbs/ Kitchen Aids
Low blood sugar	Iron herbs, ferric phosphate (cell salt #4)	Oil of sassafras: Rub in 3 drops on the sole of each foot twice daily for 4 weeks.
Low vitality		12-herb tincture formula[1]
LSD, overdose/residue		Chaparral: Take in tablet form.
Lumbago	B-complex, B_1	
Lung, abscesses		Cucumber juice
Lung, congestion		Fenugreek relieves congestion. Thyme tea: Relieves shortness of breath. Water: Aerate pure water by beating it with an eggbeater. Drink it at once.
Lung, cough (phlegm)		Lugworm tea: Drink 1 to 4 cups daily.
Lung, diseases		Cabbage is anti-inflammatory and antibacterial. Cardamom has a soothing effect on membranes and lungs. Add dill to your food. Eat fish, vegetables, salads, very few carbohydrates, and lots of cream, fat, or butter.
Lung, strengthener		Calamus root

[1] The herbs include apple tree bark, calamus root, burdock root, pimpernel root, angelica root, cherry bark, rhubarb root, gentian root, aloes, cascara sagrada bark, nutmeg, and myrrh.

HEALTH ISSUE | | REMEDIES
| Vitamins/
Minerals | Spices/Herbs/
Kitchen Aids

Health Issue	Vitamins/Minerals	Spices/Herbs/Kitchen Aids
Lung, weak		Lugworm tea: Drink 1 to 4 cups daily
Lupus (skin)		*Thuja occidentalis* (homeopathic) Bring wine vinegar to a boil and thicken it with barley flour. Apply to skin.
Lymph cleanser		Barley: Boil 3 tbls. in 1 quart water for 30 minutes. Strain. Add a little clove and cinnamon. Drink this in 1 day. It will clear congestion in the lymphatic system.
Lymph glands, diseased		Echinacea: 2 capsules or more daily for 3 days.
Lymph glands, enlarged		Pokeroot tea
Lymph glands, swollen		Lettuce; basil
Lymphatic system	Potassium	Cucumber: Four or 5 cups of cucumber juice a day for 1 week purifies the lymphatic system and the blood and clears the complexion. Bananas keep lymphatic system fit.
Lymphatic trouble		Burdock root tea: Drink 2 cups daily.
Magnetism, increase in		Mistletoe (*Viscum album*) (homeopathic)
Malaria		Collard seed, parsley seed, red pepper seed

HEALTH ISSUE	REMEDIES	
	Vitamins/ Minerals	Spices/Herbs/ Kitchen Aids
Maliciousness		Cashew (*Anacardium occidentale*) (homeopathic)
Mammary glands, underdeveloped		Saw palmetto (Sabal serrulate) (homeopathic)
Mania		Horsetail
Marrow of bones, strengthener		Yarrow tea
Measles	C, minerals from raw potatoes (grated)	First stage: Eyebright Later stage: Wind flower (*Pulsatilla*) (homeopathic); Alfalfa seeds; Linden blossoms
Meditation, aid for deeper		Lavender tea
Melancholy		Basil: Keep in open bowl in the room to dispel melancholy, for the aroma tends to make people happy. Also season food with it. Club moss (*Lycopodium clavatum*) (homeopathic) Vanilla bean: Cut 1 bean into pieces and boil in 1 pint of water. Drink 6 ozs. 2 or 3 times daily.
Memory		Almonds: Take 6 to 10 a day. Almond oil: Take 1 tsp. a day. Cloves: 4 cloves in any tea mixture, daily. Eyebright tablets Mustard seeds: 2 seeds for memory.

HEALTH ISSUE REMEDIES

	Vitamins/ Minerals	Spices/Herbs/ Kitchen Aids
Memory (cont.)		Prunes: Take 3 daily. Rosemary tea Sage: On a slice of buttered rye bread. Ginkgo biloba
Men, developing female breasts	B (estrogen gets upset with lack of B_1)	
Ménière's disease (see also Inner ear)	B-complex, B_6, B_1, B_{12}, C, E, F, niacin, potassium, bioflavonoids	
Meningitis		Aloe vera leaves: Take a couple, about 6 inches long, and wash and cut into small pieces. Add 3 times the amount of water and simmer for 10 minutes. Add 2 tbls. honey or more to taste and simmer for another 5 minutes. Cool, strain, and give 1 tbl. to adult every hour, and 1 tsp. to a child every hour. The sicker you are, the smaller the dosage. Goldenseal, skullcap: Make tea to use for enemas.
Menopause	Calcium, magnesium, red bone marrow B-complex: A high potency taken 1 to 3 times daily further supports the nervous system, and a daily intake of vitamin E has been known to eliminate hot flashes and night sweats.	

Health Issue	Remedies	
	Vitamins/ Minerals	Spices/Herbs/ Kitchen Aids
Menopause (cont.)	Vitamin D: Needed in adequate amounts or a deficiency causes nervousness, irritability, and headaches. Depression and arthritic problems may develop.	Black cohosh: in capsules. Rue tea: 2 cups daily. Yarrow: in capsules. Cinnamon, yams also beneficial.
Menses, regulator		Wind flower (*Pulsatilla*) (homeopathic)
Menstrual cramps, relieved		Lemon balm, motherwort, oregano help relieve cramps. Cramp bark: 1 cup tea as needed.
Menstrual difficulties		Blue cohosh: 2 capsules needed.
Menstrual flow, excessive	B-complex, B_{12}, E, folic acid, iron, trace minerals from okra	Okra Shepherd's purse tea: 2 cups daily
Menstrual flow, irregular	B-complex, E, folic acid, sulfur, trace minerals from fireweed	
Menstrual flow, promotes		Motherwort tea Hot ginger tea: stimulates delayed menses; relieves cramps.
Menstrual flow, scanty		Thyme tea
Menstruation, clots		Shepherd's purse: 2 cups daily, 1 tsp. to 1 cup of boiling water.
Menstruation, disturbed due to emotion		Tiger Lily (*Lilium tigrinum*) (homeopathic)

HEALTH ISSUE   REMEDIES

	Vitamins/ Minerals	Spices/Herbs/ Kitchen Aids
Menstruation, PMS (see Premenstrual syndrome)		
Mental buoyancy		Take alfalfa seed tea or in tablet form.
Mental depression	Sodium	Cleavers tea
Mental dullness	Iodine	Hawthorn tea or in tablet form. Eyebright, dulse: Equal parts and make tea.
Mental exhaustion	Lecithin	Sage
Mental health		Iodine herbs (see chapter 16)
Mental instability		Agar, sorrel: Make tea and drink.
Mental strength		Iodine herbs (see chapter 16)
Mental upset		Meadowsweet tea: 2 cups daily.
Mentally hard to please	Iron	
Mercury in tissues	Selenium containing colloidal minerals is effective in removing mercury.	Emu-mu (oil made from the emu bird and other special oils) counteracts mercury in the nervous system.
Metallic poison (see also Poison, metals)	Vitamin C	Pumpkin seed, okra, rhubarb root, capsicum, peppermint, dulse (herbal formula)

HEALTH ISSUE	REMEDIES	
	Vitamins/ Minerals	Spices/Herbs/ Kitchen Aids
Metallic poison (cont.)		Green beans and zucchini: Eat exclusively for 3 days; will get rid of metallic poison. Squash and strawberries: Removes arsenic poison. Extra good for smokers. It also removes other metallic poisons. Vitamin C, squash, Mexican raw sugar: 1 tsp. several times daily until symptoms subside. Wheat sprouts: Improve detoxification of tissues; protect against heavy metal damage in the body.
Migraine (see also Headache)		Blue vervain (*Verbena hastata*) tea At the start of a headache: Brazilian cocoa (guarana) Lavender oil: Apply on forehead. A specific homeopathic remedy for dioxin
Milk allergy		Parsnips: Boil in plenty of water; blend to a smooth pulp. When sensitive to milk products, take 1 to 2 tsps. of parsnip pulp before drinking milk.
Milk leg		Cayenne, externally
Mineral supplier		Alfalfa seeds: Use as sprouts, tea, or tablets.

HEALTH ISSUE	REMEDIES	
	Vitamins/ Minerals	Spices/Herbs/ Kitchen Aids
Miscarriage		Rosemary can help prevent miscarriage. Apple tree bark tea will check miscarriages.
Mononucleosis	B-complex, B_6, C, E, pantothenic acid, copper, trace minerals from lettuce water and raspberry leaf tea	Red raspberry leaf tea Leaf lettuce water/tea Apply raw tomato poultices to the neck for swelling.
Moodiness	Sulfur	Mallow leaf tea
Morning sickness (see also Pregnancy)	B_6 and trace minerals from peach leaf tea	Peach leaf tea
Morphine habit		Oats Celery root (celeriac)
Mosquito bite		Bar soap: Moisten a little and rub over bite. It will stop itching. Mix baking soda and cream of tartar with a bit of water to make a paste. Apply to bite.
Mother, healthy		Squaw vine Raspberry leaf tea: 2 cups daily.
Mother, nursing (see Nursing, pain)		
Mother's milk, drying up		Cranesbill (strong tea): Massage into breasts. Sage tea: Drink 3 cups a day.

HEALTH ISSUE | REMEDIES

	Vitamins/ Minerals	Spices/Herbs/ Kitchen Aids
Mother's milk, increasing		Caraway: 1 tsp. caraway seed in 8 oz. cold water. Bring to a boil, simmer for a few minutes, and drink several cups a day to increase mother's milk. Fennel seed in barley water. Alfalfa, blessed thistle Lentils
Motion sickness	B_6	Cover solar plexus with newspaper. In less than 10 minutes, relief.
Mouth		Nutmeg: Take when tongue adheres to the roof of the mouth. Savory: Excellent antiseptic mouthwash and gargle.
Mouth, burning		Poppy seed (available in your spice section): Make tea. Hold in your mouth several times a day.
Mouth, dry		Chew cloves or calamus root.
Mouth, odor		Chew juniper berries, caraway seed, or parsley leaves. Gargle rosemary tea.
Mouth, ulcers	Zinc (when corners of mouth are cracked)	Chew sage or willow leaves. Hold blackberry leaf tea in mouth. Myrrh

HEALTH ISSUE	REMEDIES	
	Vitamins/ Minerals	Spices/Herbs/ Kitchen Aids
Mouth, ulcers (cont.)		Carrots: Grated, wrapped in a cloth and applied to canker sores. Change every 2 hours.
Mucous		Oranges: Cleansers of the stomach, ears, head, and sinuses if taken in the following manner: Drink 1 glass of fresh-squeezed juice followed by the same amount of distilled water. DO NOT MIX. Do this as often as you want, 10 times daily or so. NO OTHER FOODS should be taken for 2 days. Do this 2 days in a row, 3 times a year.
Mucous, solvent		Fenugreek; Southernwood In bronchi, rattling: garlic In lungs: Calamus root tea
Multiple sclerosis	B-complex, E, C, B, B_{15}, lecithin, niacin, magnesium, pantothenic acid	Combine corn, grated carrots, liquid garlic, chives, milk, dry mustard, paprika, flaxseed oil, and primrose oil. Place all in a blender; add salt or pepper to taste. Emu-mu drops (oil made from the emu bird and other special oils) help rebuild the central nervous system. Make tea of sunflower and fenugreek seeds: Drink 1 cup 3 times daily. Pineapple and avocado Thyme tea

HEALTH ISSUE	REMEDIES	
	Vitamins/ Minerals	Spices/Herbs/ Kitchen Aids
Mumps		Linden flower bath: Take a handful of flowers, brew, strain, and add to bath. Pokeroot tea: 1 cup 3 times daily
Mumps, after second stage		Wind flower (*Pulsatilla*) (homeopathic) Gotu kola Linden blossom tea
Mumps, residue		Gotu kola: In capsules
Muscle, aches in shoulder	Magnesium	
Muscle, builders		Beans and corn: Use in various combinations, such as beans and cornbread or corn tortillas and beans. Rye
Muscle, calves very tense		Chickpea (*Lathyrus sativus*) (homeopathic)
Muscle, cramps	B_1, B_2, E, calcium lactate	
Muscle, deterioration		Shepherd's purse tea: Drink 2 cups daily.
Muscle, function	E	
Muscle, jerks	Magnesium needed	
Muscle, pain	B, E, calcium lactate	Rub a piece of raw potato over the muscle.
Muscle, spasms (daytime)	Magnesium	Marjoram

HEALTH ISSUE   REMEDIES

	Vitamins/ Minerals	Spices/Herbs/ Kitchen Aids
Muscle, spasms (evening)	Calcium lactate	Marjoram
Muscle, strength		Buckwheat: Use in pancakes, cereal, or main dishes. Chia seed: Soak 1 tsp. seed in 4 ozs. of juice for 2 to 3 hours and drink this 3 to 4 times a day.
Muscle, tendon and tissue injuries		Apply comfrey root compresses. Arnica tincture: A few drops in water, make compress. Also put a few drops in water and drink. Daisy tea: Drink 2 to 3 cups daily. Lady's mantle (*Alchemilla vulgaris*)
Muscle, twitching		Skullcap
Muscle, weakness	Potassium	Apple peelings: Take a handful of peelings, boil them for 20 minutes in 1 quart water. Strain and take 6 ozs. daily. Gentian tea: ½ cup twice daily. Jerusalem artichokes Sesame seeds: Complete amino acid supplier. Supply osmium, a trace mineral. Shepherd's purse Wormwood with lady's mantle tea.

HEALTH ISSUE	REMEDIES	
	Vitamins/ Minerals	**Spices/Herbs/ Kitchen Aids**
Muscle, weakness after illness		Almonds: Eat alone or add to food.
Muscle, weakness in children		Barley malt Juniper berry branches: Boil for 45 minutes, strain, and add the tea to bathwater. Soak for 20 minutes.
Muscle, weakness in the elderly		Yarrow tea: 2 cups daily.
Muscular dystrophy	A, B_6, B_{12}, E, C, B-complex, choline, inositol, pantothenic acid	
Myopic astigmatism		Tiger lily (*Lilium tigrinum*) (homeopathic)
Nails	A, calcium, B_2	
Narcotic poisoning		Bayberry tea or in capsules.
Nausea		Flowers and oil of cloves. Nutmeg, peppermint, lemon balm, ginger, clove, and cinnamon relieve nausea. Peach leaf tea (if constant) Summer savory: ½ tsp.
Nearsightedness	A, B-complex, C, E	
Neck, aching	Magnesium	Watch for reproductive organs out of harmony.

HEALTH ISSUE	REMEDIES	
	Vitamins/ Minerals	Spices/Herbs/ Kitchen Aids
Neck, pain		Comfrey root tea Rose petals Red clover tops Orange blossoms, nutmeg, mace
Neck, stiff (see Stiff, neck)		
Needles and pins	B_{12}, folic acid	
Nephritis	A, B_2, B_6, choline, inositol, lecithin, calcium, magnesium, potassium, trace minerals from herb teas	Watermelon seed tea
Nephritis, acute		Elder flower tea: Drink 4 cups daily.
Nerve food	Vitamin C	Apple whey: Take 1 pint apple juice or apple wine, 1 pint water, 1 pint milk. Heat it slowly, but do not bring to a boil. When it curdles, strain it through fine cloth. Throw curds away, sweeten with honey if needed. Take 2 tbls. 5 times daily if person is very weak. Appetite will improve and all signs of illness will disappear. As patient grows stronger, increase to 2 cups a day. Cherry juice, egg yolk: Add egg yolk to a 6-ounce glass of cherry juice, stir, and drink. Egg yolk: Two yolks from good healthy eggs mixed with 4 oz. grape juice once or twice daily.

HEALTH ISSUE	REMEDIES	
	Vitamins/ Minerals	Spices/Herbs/ Kitchen Aids
Nerve food (cont.)		Pineapple juice, prune juice: Combined, rebuilds exhausted nerves. Take 6 ozs. 3 times daily. Strawberries: Rich in vitamin C and minerals. Especially good for nervous disorders and to help build up weak kidney and bladder. Eat 4 ozs. 2 times daily.
Nerves (see also Sedatives)		Almonds: Blanch with grapes. Celery: Eat crisp and tender celery for depleted nerves. Lavender: In bathwater. Lily, green leaves: Tie on painful spots. Place a red and green towel in your bed. Sleep on it. Sage: In bathtub and as tea. St. John's wort oil: On painful spots.
Nerves, in knots		Lily oil
Nerves, inflamed/ infected (very painful)		Peppermint tea Peppermint lotion: Apply locally.
Nerves, injuries		Daisy tea: Drink 2 to 3 cups daily.
Nerves, involuntary nervous system		Two-thirds of all nerve diseases are related to kidney trouble. Ginseng Horsetail tea

HEALTH ISSUE	REMEDIES	
	Vitamins/ Minerals	Spices/Herbs/ Kitchen Aids
Nerves, pain in arms and legs		Yarrow tea: 1 handful yarrow, brewed, strained, and added to bath.
Nerves, sedative		Myrtle tea
Nerves, tonic		Oat water: Add to fruit juice. Barley water: Add to fruit juice.
Nervous, conditions		Motherwort tea: 2 cups daily. Valerian root: ½ cup twice daily. Hops, St. John's wort, rosemary: Mix, make tea, and drink 2 cups daily. Caraway mixed with anise Bugleweed tea; Sage tea
Nervous disorders		Onion: Poultice applied to calves of legs does wonders. Marjoram Many nerve diseases have kidney trouble.
Nervous exhaustion	Silicon herbs	
Nervous heart palpitation	B-complex, B_6, lecithin, magnesium, calcium, trace minerals from valerian root	Rue tea (DO NOT take during pregnancy)
Nervous system, involuntary		Horsetail tea Ginseng

HEALTH ISSUE	REMEDIES	
	Vitamins/ Minerals	Spices/Herbs/ Kitchen Aids
Nervous tension		Catnip, mint: Make tea and drink 1 cup as needed.
Nervous weakness, after illness		Skullcap tea: ½ cup 3 times daily.
Nervousness	Magnesium, lecithin, calcium, B-complex, B_6	Mix hops, St. John's wort, and rosemary. Make a tea and drink 2 cups a day.
Neuralgia	B-complex	Allspice: Boil crushed fruit and apply on a cloth. St. John's wort (*Hypericum perforatum*) (homeopathic) Primrose Passion flowers: 2 cups daily. Salt: Heat in frying pan or oven. Put in a cloth bag and apply to painful face. White beet: Boil and apply small poultice sack to the painful area. Mullein oil, yarrow oil, chamomile oil, thyme oil: Mix the oils and apply to pain. Chamomile tea Red onion: Use as a poultice. In ankle: Mullein In right ankle: Yarrow In lower jaw: Prickly ash; raw plantain juice over painful area.
Neurasthenia		Gentian tea: Drink ½ cup twice daily.

HEALTH ISSUE — REMEDIES

	Vitamins/ Minerals	Spices/Herbs/ Kitchen Aids
Neuritis, eye	B-complex, B_1	
Neuritis, from arsenic poison	B_6, niacin	
Neuritis, from alcohol, lead, drug poison	B-complex, B_6, niacin, trace minerals from okra, pumpkin	Okra, pumpkin
Neuritis, lower extremities	B_6, niacin, B-complex	
Neuritis, unknown cause	B-complex, B_1, B_{15}, B_6, B_{12}, lecithin, pantothenic acid, C-complex	Combine avocado with agar-agar (dry), lime juice, and raw rolled oats. Drink plenty of distilled water between meals.
Neurotic, loss of power		Saw palmetto
Nibbling habit		Alfalfa tablets Barberry tea: ½ cup 3 times daily.
Night blindness	Vitamin A	Club moss tea: 1 cup
Night sweats, profuse		Dandelion leaf tea: 3 cups Linden blossom tea
Nightmares		Rosemary: A sprig under the pillow has been known to alleviate children's nightmares.
Noise, distraction by	B-complex, calcium, magnesium	*Nux vomica* (homeopathic)
Nose, bleed	C, bioflavonoids, B_{15}, B-complex, iron, K_2 from alfalfa, trace minerals from okra	Shepherd's purse: 2 cups daily.

HEALTH ISSUE   REMEDIES

	Vitamins/ Minerals	Spices/Herbs/ Kitchen Aids
Nose, blowing frequently		Couch grass tea: 2 tbls. to 1 cup of water. Drink several cups daily.
Nose, chronic nasal inflammation		Bloodroot tea: ½ cup 2 times daily.
Nose, crusts forming in	Calcium fluoride	
Nose, dry and obstructed		Elder flower tea: 2 cups daily. Put arms in warm bath. Add sage to the water. Also boil basil in milk and steep a tsp. of sage in it. Drink 6 oz. a day. Sage boiled in milk, 2 tbls. several times a day.
Nose, polyps		A strong tea made of oak bark, sniffed up the nose several times daily. Dulcamara roots made in tea and sniffed several times a day.
Nose, redness		Wash with a borax solution and rub strawberries over it.
Numbness, in fingertips and tongue, lower lip		Chickpea (*Lathyrus sativus*) (homeopathic) Anise tea: For lower lip.
Nursing pain (goes from nipple all over body)		Pokeroot tea: 2 cups daily.
Obesity (see also Antifat; Overweight)		Celery: A low-calorie reducing aid. Celery seed: Drink the tea.

HEALTH ISSUE   REMEDIES

	Vitamins/ Minerals	Spices/Herbs/ Kitchen Aids
Obesity (cont.)		Fennel: Use seeds or entire plant.
Odors, cannot bear		*Nux vomica* (homeopathic)
Old age		12-herb tincture formula[1] Primrose flowers Sage: Drink 1 cup of sage tea after each meal. Or take one slice of whole-grain bread, butter it, and sprinkle generously with sage. After eating this all weariness is gone. Sauerkraut: Keeps old age diseases away, such as stiffness, failing eyesight, wrinkles, constipation, and general useless feelings.
Optic nerves		Tomato: Leaves or peelings—do not boil; cover leaves with hot water. Let stand 15 minutes, drain, and set in refrigerator. Dosage: 1 tsp. 3 times daily before meals.
Osmium supplier		Sesame seeds: Make strong-willed people and prevent nervous breakdown. Also, squash, raspberries, and Indian corn are good osmium suppliers.
Osteoarthritis (see also Pituitary, deficiency)	B-complex, B_1, B_{12}, B_{15}, C, E, bioflavonoids, bonemeal for calcium	Can be helped by feeding the pituitary gland.

[1] The herbs include apple tree bark, calamus root, burdock root, pimpernel root, angelica root, cherry bark, rhubarb root, gentian root, aloes, cascara sagrada bark, nutmeg, and myrrh.

HEALTH ISSUE   REMEDIES

	Vitamins/ Minerals	Spices/Herbs/ Kitchen Aids
Osteoporosis	B-complex, B_{12}, C, D, calcium, magnesium, phosphorus, bonemeal and kelp for trace minerals	Kelp Bonemeal
Otitis (inflammation of ear)		Wind flower (*Pulsatilla*) (homeopathic)
Ovarian cyst		Calendula (2 parts), yarrow (1 part), nettle (1 part): Mix and make tea using 2 tbls. to 1 quart of water. Drink 1 quart daily for 4 weeks.
Ovaries, lump in		Calendula (2 parts), plantain (1 part), yarrow (1 part): Make and drink tea. One quart daily for 4 weeks.
Ovaries, swollen	Potassium, trace minerals from fire weed	
Ovaries, weak	B-complex, C-complex, copper, iron, silicon	
Overweight (see also Antifat; Obesity; Reducing)	B-complex, C, pantothenic acid, potassium from apple vinegar, glycine	Celery seed; fresh celery; lady's mantle Chickweed tea: 4 cups daily. Cleavers: 2 cups daily. Raspberry leaf tea: 1 cup 3 times daily. Fennel seed tea: Simmer 1 tsp. in 8 oz. water for 10 minutes. Drink 3 to 4 cups a day. To reduce: Angelica (2 parts), caraway (1 part).

HEALTH ISSUE   REMEDIES

	Vitamins/ Minerals	Spices/Herbs/ Kitchen Aids
Overweight (cont.)		To stimulate glands: 2 tbls. kelp. Take 1 tsp. gelatin (contains glycine) with each meal.
Overwork	B-complex, C, pantothenic acid	
Pain, burning	B_{12}, folic acid	
Pain, facial muscle	B_{12}, folic acid	
Pain, fingertips, head, and heels	Iron	Alfalfa (releases pain in head and limbs) Blue flag (*Iris versicolor*) (homeopathic) (for head pain with nausea) Lady's slipper tea, lavender tea, lavender oil applied to temples (for nerve pain in head) St. John's wort (for pain in Achilles tendon)
Pain, general		Aconite (*Aconitum napellus*), comfrey (*Symphytum officinale*), chicory (*Chichorium intybus*), black bryony (*Tamus communis*) Echinacea: For pain of a wandering nature. Epsom salts: Pour 3 lbs. in bath and soak for ½ hour until pain recedes. Lavender: In bags, applied hot, will quickly relieve almost any localized pain. Pokeroot tea: For shifting pain.

HEALTH ISSUE	REMEDIES	
	Vitamins/ Minerals	Spices/Herbs/ Kitchen Aids
Pain, general (cont.)		Salt: Heat in a frying pan, put in cloth sack, and place on painful area; cover with hot water bottle. Strawberries: Contain organic salicylates (active ingredient in aspirin). Yams: For any kind of pain.
Pain, hands and feet		Epsom salt: Put 1 tbl. in warm water; soak approx. 20 minutes.
Pain, shoulder-arm syndrome (see also Shoulder)	Iron, copper, B$_{12}$, folic acid	Echinacea tea or in capsules: For pectoral muscles.
Pain, stump (amputated leg)	B$_1$, B$_{12}$	
Painful breathing	Iron	
Painful piles	Silicon	
Palsy		Onion: Eat 1 raw daily.
Pancreas	Iodine: 1 drop in glass of water for trouble that can be detected by the sense of oppression in the stomach region.	Calamus root: Chew the root. Nutmeg: Use freshly ground and store it only briefly, for it becomes rancid easily and does not work. Take ½ tsp. in hot water to stimulate liver/pancreas. Red beets
Pancreas, food		Green beans: Boil in plenty of water until done.

	Vitamins/ Minerals	Spices/Herbs/ Kitchen Aids
Pancreas, food (cont.)		Drink the bean water, 1 cup daily, and eat 1 cup of cooked green beans daily to strengthen the pancreas. Leeks: Use in soups and salads, steamed or boiled. Leeks stimulate insulin production. Stewed tomatoes: Cleanse the pancreas.
Pancreas, weak		Blue flag (*Iris versicolor*) (homeopathic)
Pancreatic flukes		A specific homeopathic remedy for pancreatic flukes.
Pancreatitis		Blueberries and bananas
Paralysis, facial muscles	B_{12}, folic acid	Left side: Prickly ash tea—1 cup twice daily. Stroke: Tobacco water—Wash limbs with tobacco water. Tongue: Prickly ash—Chew herb.
Paralysis, muscle	pantothenic acid	Lavender oil (not to be taken internally) is of service when rubbed on externally for stimulation of paralyzed limbs. Applied hot, it will relieve almost any local pain. Lavender tea is excellent for relieving headaches due to fatigue. Also, lavender oil rubbed on temples will help relieve headache.

Health Issue	Remedies	
	Vitamins/ Minerals	Spices/Herbs/ Kitchen Aids
Parasites		Apple cider vinegar: Take 2 tsps. every day in 6 to 7 oz. water.
		Cloves, pumpkin, and pumpkin seeds also help rid body of worms/parasites.
		For tapeworm: Take 5 parts juniper berries and 5 parts white oil for one day. (Pomegranate is also helpful.)
		Garlic: Take 3 cloves of garlic and boil in 1 cup milk for 5 minutes. Cool and strain; drink every night for 10 nights in a row.
		Lima bean pods and peach tree leaves alleviate microscopic parasites.
		Thyme: Used to treat roundworms, tapeworms, threadworms, and hook-worms.
		Calcera carbonica (homeo-pathic)
Parkinson's disease		Emu oil removes blockage from the central nervous system in a short time.
Pectoral muscle, pain		Echinacea tea or in capsules
Pelvic portal, circulation to		Tansy tea: ½ cup twice daily.
Pep drink (see also Booster)		Combine: 3 cups pine-apple juice, 1 cup water, 1 cup alfalfa sprouts, 10 almonds, or 2 cups pineapple juice.

HEALTH ISSUE	REMEDIES	
	Vitamins/ Minerals	Spices/Herbs/ Kitchen Aids
Pep drink (cont.)		Take 2 tbls. seeds and dates and blend with 8 to 10 oz. water.
Pepsin, lack of		Hops tea: Before meals.
Pepsin supplier		Pineapple juice: Take 2 ozs. before meals.
Perspiration		To encourage: Drink Linden flower tea, hot lemonade.
Phlebitis (see also Varicose veins)	C, E, bioflavonoids, trace minerals from white oak bark tea	Witch hazel; Stone root (*Collinsonia canadensis*) Reduce salt; Reduce meat Black radish root, parsley leaves (herbal formula) Goldenseal root capsule: 1 every hour. Use cottage cheese compresses. White oak bark tea: 1 to 2 quarts.
Photophobia	A, B$_2$	
Pigmentation of skin	A, C, E	
Piles, painful	Silicon herbs, B$_6$	Dates and milk instead of breakfast.
Pimples (see also Acne; Boils and pimples)		Lemon verbena tea: Dampen a clean cloth and scrub face vigorously. Repeat for 9 days and see an improvement. Epsom salts: Make a brine and pat on the face with

Health Issue	Remedies	
	Vitamins/ Minerals	Spices/Herbs/ Kitchen Aids
Pimples (cont.)		cotton. Let dry before going to bed. Do this until pimples are dried up.
Pinkeye		Potato: Raw, grated potatoes over closed eye. Or take thin slices of raw potato and cover eye. It will release pain, and the redness will go away. Red potatoes are best. Soak a clean cloth in warm water and apply to the eyes a few minutes several times a day. Be sure to wash anything that comes in contact with your eyes. See a doctor if it doesn't clear up in a few days.
Pituitary, deficiency		Alternate: 1 bunch of watercress one day, and 6 oz. pineapple juice 2 times the next day. Cherry bark, Cherry juice Wild cherry bark tincture: 7 drops twice daily.
Pleurisy		Flaxseed: As tea and as poultice. Lady's mantle tea: 2 cups daily. Pleurisy root tea: Several cups. Thyme, fennel: Make tea. This combination relaxes.
Pneumonia		Cranberry juice: Preferred over any other juice. Collard seeds, parsley seeds, spinach seeds,

HEALTH ISSUE   REMEDIES

	Vitamins/ Minerals	Spices/Herbs/ Kitchen Aids
Pneumonia (cont.)		onion seeds: Simmer 1 tsp. of each of the seeds in 1 pint water. One pint water needs 4 tbls. of seeds. Drink 4 oz. every hour. Milk: Warm milk compresses around the upper torso. Take a towel, did in warm milk, wrap around body. Wrap with plastic, then warm cloth. Also, hold right hand over forehead and left hand on lower back of head for 20 minutes.
Poison ivy		Epsom salts: Wet Epsom salts and apply to painful areas. Fels Naphtha soap: Wash with Fels naphtha soap— no more trouble. White oak bark tea bath; Sassafras tea bath; Tansy tea bath; *Rhus toxicodendron* (homeopathic)
Poison, metals (see also Metallic poison)		Combine: 2 tbls. ground pumpkin seeds, 1 tbl. okra powder, ½ tsp. cayenne pepper. When mixed take 1 tsp. of this in 1 tbl. rhubarb sauce about 3 times a day for 10 days. A universal remedy for removing lead, arsenic, platinum, gold, and mercury from your body.
Poison oak		White oak bark tea: Apply.

HEALTH ISSUE REMEDIES

	Vitamins/ Minerals	Spices/Herbs/ Kitchen Aids
Poison oak (cont.)		Rub cream of tartar over the area. Homeopathic Anacardium is an antidote.
Poisons, flushing from system		Combine anise and caraway: Make tea and drink 3 cups a day.
Poisons, swallowed		Charcoal: It will absorb up to ½ its weight in poison. Burn a piece of bread, toasting it many times.
Poliomyelitis		Chickpea (*Lathyrus sativus*) (homeopathic)
Pollution		Willow leaf tea: 2 cups daily.
Polyneuritis, of toxic nature	B-complex, B_6, B_{12}, C	
Polyps	A, silicon	For the mouth: Horsetail. For the nose: Oak bark tea (strong). Sniff it into nose several times daily.
Poor equilibrium	Iron, B-complex, C	
Potassium, lack of		Lady's mantle; Banana
Pregnancy		Coconut milk: Pregnant women should take this regularly in the morning on an empty stomach. It will brings clear urine and also nourish the fetus. The child will be a healthy one.

| HEALTH ISSUE | REMEDIES | |
	Vitamins/ Minerals	Spices/Herbs/ Kitchen Aids
Pregnancy (cont.)		Ginger: Relieves morning sickness. Peaches: A complete food for mother and fetus. Also, drink peach leaf tea for morning sickness.
Premenstrual syndrome (PMS)	Calcium, magnesium	Cramp bark tea: 1 cup as needed. Black cohosh Feed the adrenal glands.
Premenstrual tension	A	
Prevention, AIDS		Take 1 tbl. lecithin granules and 1 egg yolk (fresh), mix thoroughly and add to juice (no citrus), water, or skim milk. Do this twice a week. This will liquefy the virus so it cannot attach.
Prevention, colds		Thyme tea: 1 cup daily, 1 tsp. to 1 cup; feeds the thymus gland.
Prevention, infectious diseases		Pimpernel or juniper berries: This was used to prevent the plague in the Middle Ages.
Prevention, mosquito bites	B_1, B_6	
Prolapsed organs		Lady's mantle tea: Drink 3 or 4 cups daily; 1 tsp. per 1 cup of boiling water.
Prolapsed womb		Squawroot, life root: 1 tsp. 5 times daily.

HEALTH ISSUE   REMEDIES

	Vitamins/ Minerals	Spices/Herbs/ Kitchen Aids
Prostate, enlarged	A, B-complex, C, E, F, potassium, trace minerals from fenugreek tea	Couch grass Echinacea: 2 capsules 3 times daily. Milk compresses: Make as you would give a diaper to a baby. Warm the milk (Do Not Boil), soak a Turkish or terry cloth towel (cotton) in it and apply as a diaper. Cover with a hot water bottle and place a plastic sheet underneath.
Prostate, general health	Zinc	Coconut: Coconut milk is a specific for toning up the prostate gland. An herbal combination of tansy, clay, milkweed, cramp bark, goldenseal leaves, and blessed thistle, along with an herbal combination of black walnut leaves, saw palmetto berries, and cornsilk. Myrrh: Cleanses the system Pumpkin seed; Saw palmetto tincture; Bee pollen
Protein		Avocado: Fat and protein supplier. Lentils: Supply protein and iron of the best quality. Meat: Gives explosive energy; appetite satisfying. Millet: Vegetarian; 15 percent protein; millet is easily digested.

HEALTH ISSUE   REMEDIES

	Vitamins/ Minerals	Spices/Herbs/ Kitchen Aids
Protein digestant		Celery, basil: Aids protein digestion. It increases appetite and is good in curing mucous; therefore, it is used for rheumatic pain, gastric trouble, cold, cough, and urinary disorders. Sage tea: 1 cup twice daily.
Protein, locked		Sage tea: 1 cup twice daily.
Psoriasis	Iodine	Blue flag (*Iris versicolor*) (homeopathic) Celandine (*Chelidonium majus*) (homeopathic) Combine: Iodine (2 part, not white), castor oil (4 parts). Mix and apply to skin once daily. Cool baths with apple cider vinegar added to water. Nettle tea; Calendula tea
Puffiness, face	Iodine	
Puffiness, swelling that comes and goes (parts of body)	Calcium fluoride	
Pulse (alternates often)	Iodine	
Pus formation	A, C, calcium, sulfur	Vinegar: Take 2 tbls. vinegar, add to 1 quart water, heat, and inhale vapor for 10 minutes 3 or 4 times a day for pus formation of lungs, sinuses, and throat.

HEALTH ISSUE   REMEDIES

	Vitamins/ Minerals	Spices/Herbs/ Kitchen Aids
Putrefaction, arrest it		Charcoal; burnt toast
Pyorrhea	A, B-complex, B_6, C, bioflavonoids, niacin, calcium, potassium	Calamus root: Chew small pieces several times daily. Goldenseal, myrrh: Make tea and hold in mouth several times daily. Make your own toothpaste: Powdered calcium (bone meal is best), sage, myrrh and goldenseal (very little, for it is bitter).
Radiation	B_6 (for side effects of)	Clorox: Add 6 oz. of Clorox-brand bleach to your bath and soak for 10 to 15 minutes. Salt, baking soda: Add 1 pound of each to your bathwater and soak for 15 minutes. Seaweed: Has a neutralizing effect (so does miso soup).
Radioactive fallout		Combine: 1 tsp. baking soda, 1 tsp. sea salt, ½ tsp. cream of tartar, 1 quart water. Mix and drink 8 ozs. every 2 hours with symptoms diminishing with every dose. Combine: 1 glass cranberry juice, ½ tsp. cinnamon, ½ tsp. powdered clove, ½ tsp. cream of tartar. Willow leaf tea: Drink 2 cups or more daily when fallout is coming down. Put in bath for children and weak adults.

HEALTH ISSUE	REMEDIES	
	Vitamins/ Minerals	Spices/Herbs/ Kitchen Aids
Rattlesnake bite		Salt: Wet some and wrap arms or feet in the salt pack. Be sure the bite gets an extra dose. Then rush to physician.
Rectum, aching or prolapsed		Spikenard tea: ½ cup twice daily.
Rectum, ulcerated		Chlorophyll: Either in capsules or in liquid form.
Reducing (see also Antifat; Obesity; Overweight)		Dulse, kelp, agar-agar Leeks: Cut and boil in water. Use the water and the tougher parts in soup and the tender parts in a salad. Leeks are pancreas food, tissue builder, and brain food.
Rejuvenation (see also Aging)		12-herb tincture formula[1]
Reproductive organs, female (to strengthen)		Yarrow; Calendula; Nettle
Reproductive organs, infection		Oak bark concoction in bathwater.
Reproductive organs, itching of genitals		Wash with strong sage tea.
Reproductive organs, male (to strengthen)		Saw palmetto (*Sabal serrulata*) (homeopathic)
Resistance, low	Calcium herbs (see chapter 16)	
Resistance to disease		Thyme tea: Drink 1 cup daily.

[1] The herbs include apple tree bark, calamus root, burdock root, pimpernel root, angelica root, cherry bark, rhubarb root, gentian root, aloes, cascara sagrada bark, nutmeg, and myrrh.

Health Issue   Remedies

	Vitamins/ Minerals	Spices/Herbs/ Kitchen Aids
Respiratory ailments		Celery seed tea Hot lemon juice with honey can relieve cough and sore throats. Marjoram, violet leaves, chickweed are helpful. Thyme tea: 1 cup daily.
Restless, eye movement	Magnesium	
Restless, finger movement	Magnesium	
Restless leg syndrome	Folic acid deficiency; lack of tryptophan; E	Eat vitamin E-rich foods.
Restlessness	B-complex, B_1, B_6, calcium lactate	Nettle tea: 1 to 2 cups daily
Retina, bleeding	C, bioflavonoids, rutin, B_1	Apply raw potato compresses. Paprika (Hungarian is best): 1 tsp. on your food 3 times daily.
RH factor	B-complex, C, bioflavonoids, enzymes from raw foods	
Rheumatic fever		Apple peeling concentrate
Rheumatic muscles		Asparagus Basil: Drink as tea and/or sprinkle on an oiled cloth and apply to ache. Sawdust: Contains natural DMSO. Take pine sawdust, boil in water for 10 minutes, and place hands or feet into the warm

HEALTH ISSUE   REMEDIES

	Vitamins/ Minerals	Spices/Herbs/ Kitchen Aids
Rheumatic muscles (cont.)		mush. When there is pain in the spine, strain the mush, put in sack, and place on area.
Rheumatism	B-complex, B, B$_{15}$, C, bioflavonoids, folic acid, calcium (In many cases, but not all.)	An herbal combination of yucca, black walnut leaves, yellow dock, wormwood, and fenu- greek seed. Avocado: Combine with Agar-agar (dry), lime juice, and raw rolled oats. Drink plenty of distilled water between meals. Basil: Drink as tea and/or sprinkle on an oiled cloth and apply to ache. Chickweed (if shifting from side to side) Horsetail tea or in capsules for pain. Marjoram tea or oil in bathwater. Or put a drop of oil on the pillow to induce sleep. Oil extracted from borage seeds: Available in capsules. Oregano: Apply externally. Raw potato: Carry a raw potato in your pocket. In 1 or 2 days, it's shriveled up and smells from the poison attracted. Replace it with another potato. Rosemary: stimulates cir- culation and eases pain. Violet root: In upper part of body, right side.

HEALTH ISSUE	REMEDIES	
	Vitamins/ Minerals	Spices/Herbs/ Kitchen Aids
Rhinitis, chronic (nasal inflammation)		Bloodroot tea: ½ cup twice daily
Rickets	D, C, calcium, kelp baths	
Ringworm (tinea)		Banana peel: Rub peel on area. Bloodroot: Externally apply strong tea. Also, peel and rub on area.
Rosacea	B_{12} (red nose)	
Rough skin	Silicon	Eat silicon-rich foods such as oats and wheat bran. Eat oatmeal and rub face and arms with oat water. Wheat bran makes the skin smooth. Make a thin paste of wheat bran and apply to face, neck, and arms.
Sadness		Basil tea or sprinkle on food.
Sadness, in the morning		Club moss tea: In the morning.
Saliva, profuse flow	Calcium (for too much in throat)	Plantain Blue flag (*Iris versicolor*) (homeopathic)
Saliva, to increase		Prickly ash tea Sage: Chew leaves Cloves: Chew
Scabies		Thyme tea: Use as a skin antiseptic.

HEALTH ISSUE   REMEDIES

	Vitamins/ Minerals	Spices/Herbs/ Kitchen Aids
Scars	Calcium Vitamin E taken externally and applied to scars.	Peppermint oil: Rub on scar. Cocoa butter: Rub on scar. It has to be done consistently, twice daily. Homeopathic: *Drosera rotundifolia;* a homeopathic remedy specific for graphites
Sciatica	B-complex, B_1, B_{15}	Elderberry juice: A specific for sciatica. Elderberry tea: Also good. Fenugreek: Make poultice of hot milk and crushed seeds. Mugwort: If sciatica is worse in hot weather use this. Pinkroot, St. John's wort, cayenne pepper, black tea: Mix and drink 1 cup.
Scurvy	C, bioflavonoids	Increase green leafy vegetables and fruit intake. Dog rose (*Rosa canina*)
Seasickness		Pennyroyal: Carry it with you when traveling.
Seborrhea, on face, lips, and mouth	B_6	
Seborrheic dermatitis	A, B-complex, biotin	
Sedative (nerves)		Myrtle tea
Self-confidence, loss of		Club moss
Self-esteem, low		12-herb tincture formula[1]

[1] The herbs include apple tree bark, calamus root, burdock root, pimpernel root, angelica root, cherry bark, rhubarb root, gentian root, aloes, cascara sagrada bark, nutmeg, and myrrh.

HEALTH ISSUE	REMEDIES	
	Vitamins/ Minerals	Spices/Herbs/ Kitchen Aids
Senility		Avoid cooking in aluminum pots and pans. Medical tests reveal that people suffering from dementia diseases have abnormally high concentrations of aluminum in the brain.
Senior, cold feeling		Lemon water with honey and 2 drops of cinnamon oil. Also, boil cinnamon pieces in water for 20 minutes. Sweeten with honey.
Shingles	B-complex, B_1, B_{12}, folic acid	Homeopathic: *Arsenicum metallicum; Ranunculus bulbosus* Celery: Drink 1½ quarts celery juice daily. Epsom salts: Make a paste by adding water to achieve the right consistency, then apply frequently to the affected parts until relief is felt. Leeks: Blend some of the leaves in blender with a little water and apply to the painful area. Peppermint tea: Use as an eyewash or skin wash. Take 4 oz. witch hazel or spirit of camphor, add 8 drops of peppermint oil, shake, and apply to painful area.
Shock		Cayenne pepper in cream.

HEALTH ISSUE	REMEDIES	
	Vitamins/ Minerals	Spices/Herbs/ Kitchen Aids
Shock (cont.)		Eating oranges calms the nerves. Hypericum or St. John's wort
Shortness of breath		Red onion juice: Bring to a boil, add honey, simmer for 15 minutes. Take 1 tsp. every hour.
Shots		Suck hard candy for 30 minutes. Spit out all saliva.
Shoulder, arm syndrome (see Pain)		
Shoulder, pain		Under right shoulder: Gallbladder Under left shoulder: Stomach
Shoulder, right (pain/ stiffness to raise arm)		Pokeroot tea: 2 cups daily
Sighing	Calcium	
Sinew, tendon and joint injuries		Apply comfrey root compresses. Arnica is best.
Singing, difficulty		Sulfur herbs (see chapter 16)
Sinus	A, C, bioflavonoids	Add 1 tbl. marjoram to one tbl. butter, boil 5 minutes and strain through cloth. Rub forehead, nose, cheeks, and nostrils with it.

Health Issue	Remedies	
	Vitamins/ Minerals	Spices/Herbs/ Kitchen Aids
Sinus (cont.)		Black pepper: Take 1 tsp. honey, grind black pepper over it (it must be freshly ground), and take as needed. Garlic: Nature's antibiotic; will help fight infection. Horseradish, onion, turnips, mustard, radishes Horseradish: Take a piece of fresh horseradish or open a jar of horseradish relish and take a little piece several times a day. Sip 12 ozs. grape juice twice daily for 6 weeks.
Skin		Comfrey: Combine with any good face or hand lotion to produce a product that has been found valuable in removing various imperfections on the skin and, in some instances, will cause wrinkles to disappear. Cucumbers: Either eat or apply topically. They cool and heal the skin.
Skin, ailments		Slippery elm: Make a poultice for skin ailments such as burns, boils, and ulcers. Homeopathic: *Thuja occidentalis; Arsenicum album;* a specific homeopathic remedy for staph

HEALTH ISSUE	REMEDIES	
	Vitamins/ Minerals	Spices/Herbs/ Kitchen Aids
Skin, blemishes		Combine ⅓ tsp. ground nutmeg, 1 tsp. honey, and 4–5 oz. hot water; take 3 mornings in a row, then a 3-day break; repeat 9 times. Garlic: Rub fresh garlic cloves on skin. Soda bicarbonate: Make a small paste of spirits of camphor in soda bicarbonate, pat on area, and leave on overnight for 1 week. Do not bandage or cover for 1 week.
Skin, blood purifier		Strawberry leaves; Primrose (*Primula officinalis*); Nettle; Ground ivy
Skin, dry and chapped		Cocoa butter (1 part), glycerin (1 part), lanolin (1 part), rose water (1 part), elder flower water (1 part): Mix and apply to skin daily. Mix 3 drops lemon oil and 3 drops glycerin: Apply to chapped hands and skin.
Skin, eczema		Strawberry leaf tea Club moss behind the ear Pansy tea (for children) Evening primrose oil on joints and fingers.
Skin, infection		White pond lily: Apply to skin.

Health Issue	Remedies	
	Vitamins/ Minerals	Spices/Herbs/ Kitchen Aids
Skin, pigmentation (dirty, oily, yellowish)	Calcium fluoride	
Skin, red and scaly	A, B$_2$, lecithin	Soybean lecithin for red, itchy, scaly skin. Make a salve and apply. Also take 2 tbls.
Skin, remedies		Cucumber: Contains a hormone needed by the pancreas to produce insulin. It is specific for skin trouble. Coconut oil: Massage on scalp and all over body in summer. Applied with success on eczema, dermatitis, etc. Myrrh: Found to help athlete's foot, eczema, cracked skin, ringworm, and wrinkles.
Skin, tumorlike eruptions		Sheep sorrel: Wash skin with strong tea.
Skunk odor		Tomato juice: Wash body and cloths with ½ cup tomato juice in water and/or ½ cup ammonia in water.
Sleep, with eyes half open	Magnesium	
Sleeplessness	B$_1$, iron (for sleeplessness at night and sleepy during the day)	Anise seed: Take 1 tsp. before going to bed. Chamomile tea; lemon balm tea; alfalfa Cowslip: Sweetened with honey.

HEALTH ISSUE | REMEDIES

	Vitamins/ Minerals	Spices/Herbs/ Kitchen Aids
Sleeplessness (cont.)		Dill seeds: Simmer in olive oil and rub on forehead. Foot bath: At night, take a hot foot bath so poisons are eliminated. Rub soles of feet with a slice of lemon after foot bath. Honey and milk: Warm a cup of milk, add 1 tsp. of honey, and drink before going to bed. Laurel leaves: Place in a small bag and lay your head on it. Nutmeg tea: Use sparingly because large doses can be poisonous and can cause miscarriage. Poppy seed: Fill a small sock and lay it on your forehead.
Sleepwalking		Mugwort tea
Smoking habit		Calamus root: Found to rebuild the lungs from smoking damage. Combine 1 rounded tsp. calamus root and 1 qt. apple juice. Boil for 15 minutes, strain, and drink 6 oz., 3 times daily. Parsley, carrots, and celery protect against certain carcinogens found in tobacco smoke; help regulate prostaglandin production.
Soft bones	Calcium	

Health Issue	Remedies	
	Vitamins/ Minerals	Spices/Herbs/ Kitchen Aids
Soles of feet, itch	Silicon	
Soles of feet, pain (heat in)		Mugwort
Sore mouth	B-complex, B_{12}, phosphorus	
Sore thighs	Silicon	
Sore throat		Ginger: Chew a piece of ginger or drink ginger tea. Make tea of licorice root and hot water. Marjoram tea: Soak cotton cloth in tea and wrap around the throat. Wrap another cloth over it, making it as airtight as possible. Leave on for several hours. Myrrh: Use as a gargle. Peppermint tea
Sores, old	Calcium, sulfur, C, B-complex	Honey: Heals and disinfects. Plantain juice: Fresh on sore. Plantain tea: Drink.
Sores, open		Apply lavender tea compresses.
Sour odor	Calcium	
Spasms, bladder		Uva ursi tea: Drink 1 cup 3 times daily.
Spasms, bowels (after food)		Valerian root tea: ½ cup
Spasms, due to fallout		Cinnamon on burnt toast

HEALTH ISSUE	REMEDIES	
	Vitamins/ Minerals	Spices/Herbs/ Kitchen Aids
Speech, staggers		Nutmeg: In small amount of water.
Speaking, difficulty		Sulfur herbs (see chapter 16)
Spinal weakness		Bran: Heat bran in your oven, fill a cloth bag with the warm bran, and apply to spine.
Spine, curvature		Chlorine herbs (see chapter 16) 12-herb tincture formula[1]: Apply to spine.
Spine, pain		Pinkroot tea
Spine, trouble		Skullcap: Take 1 cup twice daily.
Spleen		Eggplant: Reduces enlarged spleen and increases red blood corpuscles and hemoglobin. Very good for anemia. Have a chiropractor release tension in the tailbone and lumbar region. St. John's wort tea and/or as a compress. Yams and beets are helpful also.
Spleen, congestion		Blue vervain (*Verbena hastata*) tea: 2 cups
Spleen, enlarged		Daisy tea, dandelion tea: Mix and drink 2 cups daily.

[1] The herbs include apple tree bark, calamus root, burdock root, pimpernel root, angelica root, cherry bark, rhubarb root, gentian root, aloes, cascara sagrada bark, nutmeg, and myrrh.

Health Issue	Remedies	
	Vitamins/ Minerals	Spices/Herbs/ Kitchen Aids
Spleen, enlarged (cont.)		Fringe tree (*Chionanthus virginicus*)(homeopathic)
Spleen, food		Okra Pumpkin seeds: Chew very well.
Spleen, obstructed		Black tea: 1 cup with a little raw honey.
Spleen, painful		Dandelion tea, sorrel tea: Mix and drink 2 cups daily.
Spleen, soothing		Inner bark of the maple tree: Make a tea.
Spleen, swollen		Pokeroot: Make a poultice. Red beets: Eat.
Spleen and liver cleanser		Combine 2 quarts concord grape juice, juice of 6 oranges, juice of 3 lemons: Cut the white of the lemon in small pieces. Boil in a little water for 10 minutes. Strain. Add water to the drink. Then take distilled water and fill the mixture to 1 gallon. This is a 1-day supply of your food-drink intake. Just 2 days of this will cleanse organs.
Splinter		Apply honey: The splinter will come to the surface. Ice cube: Freeze the area with an ice cube, then remove the splinter painlessly.

HEALTH ISSUE   REMEDIES

	Vitamins/ Minerals	Spices/Herbs/ Kitchen Aids
Splinter (cont.)		Remove at once. If too deep, apply a fresh piece of onion, tomato, or Cell Salt No. 12 (Silica).
Sprains		Daisy, lavender: For extra sore sprains, use as a compress. Ice cold water as a compress.
Sprue	A, B-complex from rice polishings, folic acid, lecithin	
Staph infection		Savory: antibacterial, antifungal, and antiviral Oxoquiniline: from the quinine tree A specific homeopathic remedy for staph
Sterility	A, B-complex, E	
Sties		Black tea (Lipton will do): Make a poultice, place moist over the eye, bandage at night.
Stiff, neck		Basil: Drink as tea or sprinkle on food. Capsicum: Use a little bit. Celandine (*Chelidonium majus*) (homeopathic): Use when the head is drawn to the left side. Check for female trouble. Chickweed: Take 2 cups daily. Cramp bark: Take 1 cup.

HEALTH ISSUE   REMEDIES

	Vitamins/ Minerals	Spices/Herbs/ Kitchen Aids
Stiff, neck (cont.)		Hawthorn: Use when the head is drawn to the right side. Motherwort: Take 1 cup daily.
Stiff, with shooting pains	B₁₂	
Stimulant		Cayenne pepper, Capsicum, Horseradish
Stitches, between the shoulder blades		Buttercup: 2 cups daily.
Stitches, in chest		Clover tea: 2 or 3 cups.
Stomach		Calamus root: uncooked Cardamom: Has a soothing effect on all membranes of the stomach and lungs. Healing to sick stomachs, ulcers, and pain: Carrot, coconut milk, eggplant, flaxseed tea, okra, parsnip, sweet potato. Indian remedy: Blackberry wine Ironweed, cashew (*Anacardium occidentale*), cleavers Persimmon: Take before meals if stomach does not behave. Unsweetened pineapple juice poured over melons develops pepsin, which is needed for digestion. Whey: Take 1 tbl. 3 times daily. This will feed the stomach glands, and they will work well again.

HEALTH ISSUE	REMEDIES	
	Vitamins/ Minerals	Spices/Herbs/ Kitchen Aids
Stomach, ache		Flaxseed: Take 2 tsps., cover with 8 ozs. boiling water, keep it warm for 30 minutes, and drink 1 to 2 cups.
Stomach, cramps		Apricot brandy: This will stop chronic stomach cramps. Take 1 tsp.
Stomach, flu		Ginger: Use ½ tsp. ground ginger to 1 cup water. Add 1 tsp. honey and drink hot. Also, hot compresses of ginger over stomach will bring relief.
Stomach, gas		Certo, apple juice: 1 tsp. Certo added to ½ glass apple juice, drink as needed.
Stomach, heaviness		Ginger tea or violet leaf tea
Stomach, sour		Raw potato slices: Eat. Charcoal tablets
Stomach, ulcers	A from carrots—carotene; B from rice polishings, E, C, bioflavonoids, K$_2$, aloe vera juice for trace minerals	Apples: Raw and cooked. Cabbage: Cabbage juice (it must be freshly made) is used for stomach ulcers because of vitamin U in cabbage. Calamus root tea: Cut root and let stand over-night in water. Then warm it (do not boil). Sip ½ cup before meals. Marigold tea, yarrow tea Okra: Cooked, do not season heavily.

HEALTH ISSUE   REMEDIES

	Vitamins/ Minerals	Spices/Herbs/ Kitchen Aids
Stomach, ulcers (cont.)		Potato: Juice 1 potato, add the same amount of warm water. Drink before each meal, 3 times a day. Red potatoes are best.
Stomach, upset		Cinnamon: Drink or chew on sticks. Pumpkin: High in beta carotene and calms upset stomach.
Stomach, weak		Gentian: Use very little. Powdered okra; Slippery elm tea; Rosemary
Stool, clay colored		Chickweed Goldenrod, goldenseal root, cloves (herbal formula)
Stool, with great force		Ground ivy tea: Drink 1 cup.
Strengthen memory	A, B-complex, C, E, pantothenic acid, silicon, glutamic acid	
Strengthen muscle	E, silicon	
Strep infection		Cucumber: Grate and squeeze the juice out. Drink 5 times a day. Chinese sumach (*Ailanthus glandulosus*) (homeopathic)
Stress	A, B-complex, B_{12}, folic acid, C, E, calcium, D, phosphorus, pantothenic acid	

| HEALTH ISSUE | REMEDIES | |
	Vitamins/ Minerals	Spices/Herbs/ Kitchen Aids
Stretch marks	E ointment	
Stroke	C, bioflavonoids, E, choline, potassium	Angelica root tea: Drink 1 cup. Lavender tea: Drink 2 cups. Mustard seed: Every morning thoroughly chew 1 tsp. Tofu: Shave head, apply tofu over head, and change the compress when tofu gets yellow.
Stroke, danger of		Rosemary
Stroke, paralysis after		Wash the limbs with tobacco water.
Stroke, tendency		Sage tea
Stuttering		Eyebright tea: Hold in mouth several times daily.
Sty		Burdock root tea: Drink it and apply. Castor oil Eyebright (*Euphrasia officinalis*) (homeopathic)
Suicidal tendencies		Black tea: Make 2 cups or more, add sugar or honey.
Summer heat		Motherwort tea
Sunburn	A, calcium without D, PABA ointment	Aloe vera Cornstarch: Mix with water to make a paste and apply to sunburn. Will ease pain.

HEALTH ISSUE | REMEDIES

	Vitamins/ Minerals	Spices/Herbs/ Kitchen Aids
Sunburn (cont.)		Lettuce leaves: Boil, strain, and let the liquid cool several hours in the refrigerator. Apply gently to sunburn.
Swelling		Adzuki beans: Boil in plenty of water. Eat them as a soup, or drink the fluid twice daily. Lettuce water: Apply externally over swollen parts of body. Raw cabbage poultice: Grate into a cheesecloth and apply overnight. Use several nights in a row for best results. Tomato: A slice on swelling reduces it quickly.
Swollen ankles	Potassium	Adzuki beans: Boil in plenty of water. Eat them as a soup or drink the fluid twice a day.
Swollen ankles and legs	Potassium	Potato peelings: Take a handful of unsprayed potato peelings and cover with 2 cups of water. Simmer 15 minutes and strain. Take 2 tbls. of this in 1 glass of water. Drink 4 glasses a day for 14 days. After several days, legs and ankles should be normal size.
Swollen glands		Baked banana skin: Mash with a little fresh cream or olive oil; make a compress. Apply.

HEALTH ISSUE   REMEDIES

	Vitamins/ Minerals	Spices/Herbs/ Kitchen Aids
Swollen knees		Raw cabbage: Grate 2 cups very fine. Wrap in cloth and apply overnight. Do several nights in a row.
Swollen ovaries	Potassium, fireweed for trace minerals	
Swollen testicles	Potassium, trace minerals from fenugreek seeds	Fenugreek seeds Echinacea: In capsule form.
Swollen toes	Iodine	
Tachycardia		Hawthorn, blessed thistle, red roses: Mix equal parts, make tea, and drink 2 cups daily.
Tapeworm		Pomegranate twigs: Boil and drink 3 cups daily during the full moon for 3 days in a row.
Tears, excessive	B_2	Basil: Place compresses over eyes.
Tears, not enough	B_1	
Teeth, clenched		Pokeroot tea: Drink 1 cup 3 times daily.
Teeth, refills (small holes)		Bone meal
Tension		Carrot seeds: Make a tea and drink a cup now and then. It will remove tension from the smooth muscles such as the intestines.

HEALTH ISSUE | | REMEDIES

Health Issue	Vitamins/ Minerals	Spices/Herbs/ Kitchen Aids
Tension, upper half of face		Violet leaf tea
Testicles, swollen (see Swollen testicles)		
Throat, dry	B_2	
Throat, lump in (globus hystericus)		Blue malva: Let sit overnight in cold water. St. Ignatius' bean (*Ignatia amara*) (homeopathic)
Throat, sore		Arnica tincture: Use 2 to 3 drops in 1 tbl. of warm water. Sage tea: Gargle Sea salt in vinegar water: Gargle.
Throat, too much saliva	Calcium	
Throat, whiter under the chin than on other parts of the neck	Manganese, sulfur	
Thrombosis	C, bioflavonoids, rutin, trace minerals from white oak bark	White oak bark tea
Thumb, drawn into the palm		Hellebore
Thymus, secretion insufficient	Copper herbs	
Thyroid, enlarged		Pokeroot compresses: Apply overnight.

HEALTH ISSUE   REMEDIES

	Vitamins/ Minerals	Spices/Herbs/ Kitchen Aids
Thyroid, sluggish	A, B-complex, C, E, choline, iodine, trace minerals from kelp (for underactive condition)	Kelp or seaweed
Tick fever		Chaparral: Take 3 tablets 3 times daily for 1 month.
Tissue	Bioflavonoid	Cabbage: Tissue builder. Leeks: Build tissue; pancreas and brain food. White of lemon: strengthens tissue. Garlic: Reduces carbohydrate residue in tissue and glands. Juniper berries: Help reduce tissue swelling. Rice: Universal acceptance by all tissues.
Tobacco, craving		Laurel leaves: Make a tea and also put in soups or meat dishes.
Toe, pain	Calcium (for cramps at night)	St. John's wort (*Hypericum perforatum*) Sour cherries: Eat 15 in the morning for 3 weeks (for gout inflammation of big toe).
Tongue, adheres to roof of mouth		Nutmeg
Tongue, burning		Blue malva tea: Boil and hold 1 tsp. in mouth.
Tongue, deep red with fissures	Niacin, B-complex	

Health Issue	Remedies	
	Vitamins/ Minerals	Spices/Herbs/ Kitchen Aids
Tongue, fissures	B$_2$	Raspberry leaf tea: Hold in mouth several times a day.
Tongue, mapped when red, scraped patches appear		Dandelion root or leaves.
Tongue, paralyzed		Ginger: Chew Lavender: Chew
Tongue, purple red	B$_2$	
Tongue, sores		Raspberry leaf tea: Hold in mouth several times daily.
Tongue, yellow or white		Peppermint leaves: Hold in mouth.
Tonic, general		Dogwood tea
Tonsils, swollen		Banana: Baked in the skin and mashed with a little fresh cream or olive oil. Make compresses. Don't eat bananas for cold or cough; they will add to the problems. Grapefruit juice Savory tea: Use as an antiseptic mouthwash and gargle.
Toothache	Magnesium (for ache when nothing is wrong)	Black tea: Soak a black tea bag in hot water, apply to cheek. Cayenne: Rub on toothache. Cloves: A little clove oil inserted into the cavity.

HEALTH ISSUE   REMEDIES

	Vitamins/ Minerals	Spices/Herbs/ Kitchen Aids
Toothache (cont.)		Powdered milk in the hole will stop the ache for a while, also.
		Hyssop: Between tooth and gum overnight.
		Oregano: Chewing on the leaf provides temporary relief.
		Pepper and mustard: Place on a piece of cloth and put over aching cheek.
Tooth, bleeding after extraction		Black tea: After extraction take one Lipton black tea bag, wet it in warm water, and apply.
Tooth, decay		Boil 1 cup of chopped mulberry bark or fine twigs in 1 quart concord grape juice for ½ hour. Take 1 tbl. 6 times daily. Keep it in your mouth, then swallow.
		Citrus fruits, licorice root extract, soy products, and curcumin prevent dental decay.
		Cheese: Eat aged cheese, such as cheddar, to prevent the formation of plaque.
Tooth, loose		Apple cider vinegar: Hold warm apple cider vinegar in your mouth, spit it out. Do this several times a day. Or boil sage with honey.
		Sage: Mix with honey and hold in mouth.

HEALTH ISSUE	REMEDIES	
	Vitamins/ Minerals	Spices/Herbs/ Kitchen Aids
Tooth, powder		Soda and salt
Tooth, strengthener		Bone meal
Toxicity	Sulfur	
Tranquilizer		Dill: Useful for its high natural mineral salt content. Sesame seeds: For sound nerves take ½ cup sesame seed, blend in 2 cups water, and add 3 tbls. whey. A little honey makes it delicious.
Tremor	Magnesium	
Trench mouth		Raspberry, oak bark: Make a juice and spray it in mouth.
Trichinosis		Oil of wintergreen (Do not take internally.)
Triglycerides, elevated		Can be a sign of diabetes or liver problems. High risk factor in cardiovascular disease and stroke. To treat: Do moderate exercise, avoid sugar, eat high-fiber diet, eliminate red meat.
Tumor		Eggplant peelings: Boil and take 2 tbls. 2 times daily. Flax oil: Use for simple tumors.

HEALTH ISSUE | | REMEDIES

Health Issue	Vitamins/ Minerals	Spices/Herbs/ Kitchen Aids
Tumor (cont.)		Tomatoes: (including juice) Contain lycopene, which is known to reduce tumors. Apply raw tomatoes to head in case of brain tumors.
		Turmeric: Use a small amount to halt tumor growth.
		Turnips: Used for deep-rooted tumors; also, deep-rooted resentments.
Tumor, fatty		Asparagus: Canned—the cheap ones are best. Blend it and take 2 tbls. in the morning and at night. Put it on bread or eat it alone.
		Bible remedy: Take 1 pound white figs in 3 quarts milk, boil until well done. Place figs in a blender, make a poultice, and apply overnight. Renew this every 12 hours for 3 days. Also, drink ½ cup of this fig milk 3 times daily.
Tumor, fibroid		Goldenrod tea
		Calendula (2 parts), yarrow (1 part), nettle (1 part): Mix and drink 1 quart daily for 4 weeks.
Tumor, ill-natured		Yellow dock, cramp bark, yarrow, milkweed, plantain, organic tobacco, tansy (herbal formula)
		12-herb tincture formula[1]; Prickly pear

[1] The herbs include apple tree bark, calamus root, burdock root, pimpernel root, angelica root, cherry bark, rhubarb root, gentian root, aloes, cascara sagrada bark, nutmeg, and myrrh.

HEALTH ISSUE	REMEDIES	
	Vitamins/ Minerals	Spices/Herbs/ Kitchen Aids
Tumor, ill-natured (breast)		Houseleek, cottonwood leaves: Make tea.
Tumor, ill-natured (female organs)		Calendula, Yarrow, Nettle
Tumor ill-natured (kidney)		Celandine (*Chelidonium majus*) (homeopathic)
Tumor, ill-natured (lip)		Juice of milkweed: Apply to lip.
Tumor, ill-natured (liver)		Calamus root: ½ cup 2 times daily. Goldenrod, goldenseal root, cloves (herbal formula)
Tumor, ill-natured (pancreas)		Calamus root: ½ cup 4 times daily. Compresses of a 12-herb tincture formula[1]
Tumor, ill-natured (stomach)		Compresses of a 12-herb tincture formula[1] Calendula, Nettle tea
Tumor, ill-natured (tongue)		Compresses of a 12-herb tincture formula[1] Celandine (*Chelidonium majus*) (homeopathic)
Tympanites (wind)		Dandelion root or leaf tea: Take after meals.
Ulcer	B-complex, B_{12}, folic acid, C, E, iron, K_2 from alfalfa	Calendula tea Calamus root: Chew Ginger: About ¼ tsp. to 6 oz. hot water relieves upset stomach.

[1] The herbs include apple tree bark, calamus root, burdock root, pimpernel root, angelica root, cherry bark, rhubarb root, gentian root, aloes, cascara sagrada bark, nutmeg, and myrrh.

HEALTH ISSUE   REMEDIES

	Vitamins/ Minerals	Spices/Herbs/ Kitchen Aids
Ulcer, duodenal		Calamus root: Let sit in cold water overnight. Warm it in the morning (do not boil). Drink ½ cup 4 to 5 times daily. Comfrey root tea: 2 cups daily. 12-herb tincture formula[1] Red potatoes
Ulcer, mouth		Sage or willow leaves Blackberry leaf tea: Hold in mouth.
Ulcer, peptic (gastric)	Vitamin U deficiency.	Thought to be cased by stress and/or dyspepsia. Treatment should include: alfalfa, cabbage juice, flax, German chamomile, and licorice. Consult physician.
Ulcer, stomach		Calamus root tea: Cut root and let stand overnight in water. Then warm it (Do Not Boil). Sip ½ cup before meals. Carrots: Cooked, relieve stomach ulcers. Fenugreek relieves ulcer of the stomach. Marigold tea; Yarrow tea; Nettle tea; Blue malva tea Red potatoes
Ulcerated colitis		Homeopathic *Thuja occidentalis*, goldenseal
Ulcerated intestines		Potatoes, garlic, goldenseal

[1] The herbs include apple tree bark, calamus root, burdock root, pimpernel root, angelica root, cherry bark, rhubarb root, gentian root, aloes, cascara sagrada bark, nutmeg, and myrrh.

HEALTH ISSUE   REMEDIES

	Vitamins/ Minerals	Spices/Herbs/ Kitchen Aids
Ulcerated rectum		Chlorophyll: Either in capsules or in liquid form.
Ulcerated skin		White pond lily Wounds: Warm milk compresses—the bacteria are drawn into the milk compresses and the infected wounds can heal.
Ulcerated stomach		Okra, apples, string beans
Ulcerated wound		Milk compresses: Draw out bacteria so wound can heal.
Urea, excessive		Senna leaf tea; Juniper berry tea; Horsetail grass tea See a physician about magnesium deficiency.
Uremia		Epsom salts drink: 1 tsp. Epsom salts in 7 ozs. water every hour for 4 hours.
Uric acid		Asparagus, cranberries, spinach, endive, and watercress: Eat 3 servings a day; must be cooked on low heat. Hydrangea (deposit) Melon: Watermelon or cantaloupe will straighten out uric acid. Sour cherries (balancer)
Urinary tract		Artichokes: Bring clear urine and are useful for albumin in the urine.

HEALTH ISSUE   REMEDIES

	Vitamins/ Minerals	Spices/Herbs/ Kitchen Aids
Urinary tract (cont.)		Celery: Increases appetite and good in curing mucous conditions, so it is used in urinary disorders. Fennel seeds with caraway seeds: Promotes the free flow of urine. Ginger: Helps in urinary difficulties.
Urination, blood in		One quart water, 4 ozs. juniper berries, boil for 10 minutes, take ½ cup 4 times daily.
Urination, burning		Marshmallow root tea: 3 or more cups as needed.
Urination, diabetic		Uva ursi tea: Drink 1 cup daily. Flaxseed tea: Drink 3 cups daily.
Urination, frequent		Cherry juice: Drink 1 glass 3 or 4 times a day.
Urination, pain with white urination		One tsp. marjoram in 8 ozs. water, simmer 10 minutes, sweeten with brown sugar. Place a handful of parsley over the bladder.
Urticaria (hives)	Niacin	Nettle, buttercup: Make tea and drink 1 cup 3 times daily.
Uterine bleeding (see also Female, bleeding)	B_6, when no other pathological disturbance can be found	Ice to nipples will stop bleeding at once.

HEALTH ISSUE	REMEDIES	
	Vitamins/ Minerals	Spices/Herbs/ Kitchen Aids
Uterus, circulation		Tansy tea: Drink ½ cup 2 times daily.
Uterus, cramps		Cramp bark tea: Drink ½ cup twice daily.
Uterus, enlarged		Yarrow tea
Uterus, prolapsed		Oak bar, squawroot, life root: Combine and make a strong tea. Take 1 tsp. 5 times daily.
Uterus, sore		Linden flower tea with honey
Vaccination, ill effects		*Thuja occidentalis* (homeopathic)
Vaginal discharge	A, B-complex, B_2, B_6, C, E, iron, trace minerals	
Varicose veins (see also Phlebitis)	Need zinc supplements.	Calendula salve: Apply. Cottage cheese compress: If possible, all night or just for several hours. Do this every night until gone. Cabbage: Grate and fill a piece of cheesecloth. Tie over painful areas and let sit overnight. (Do the same with head lettuce.) Homeopathic: *Arsenicum album*; horse chestnut (*Aesculus hippocastanum*); St. Mary's thistle (*Carduus marianus*) Marigold: 1 oz. powdered flowers and stems with 1 pint of boiling water, allow to cool and apply

HEALTH ISSUE   REMEDIES

	Vitamins/ Minerals	Spices/Herbs/ Kitchen Aids
Varicose veins (cont.)		directly to various affected parts of the body (for varicose veins, chronic ulcers, and similar ailments). Oak bark tea compress: Apply overnight. Plantain, yarrow, mullein, calendula: Mix, make tea, and drink 3 cups daily. Sage: Apply hot compresses to legs. Take frequent sage foot baths.
Varicose veins, pregnancy		Daisy tea
Varicose veins, purple		Horse chestnut
Vascular congestion		Whey: The transparent liquid released when yogurt or cheese is made. Whey removes vascular congestion and is a mind booster.
Vasodilatation		Garlic
Veins, enlarged (see also Varicose veins)		Horse chestnut
Veins, strengthener		Agrimony tea or in capsule form
Venous engorgement		Stone root (*Collinsonia canadensis*) tea: Or take 2 capsules 2 times daily.
Vermifuge (see also Parasites; Worms)		Wormwood

HEALTH ISSUE   REMEDIES

	Vitamins/ Minerals	Spices/Herbs/ Kitchen Aids
Vertigo		Crab apples: Boil and eat 1 tsp. every hour. Daisy tea (in elderly) Violet leaves
Violence		Larkspur tea: 1 tbl. 5 times daily.
Viral infection	C, bioflavonoids, A, trace minerals from sweet basil and lettuce water	Calendula tea Cinnamon, chickpeas, lettuce, basil, romaine Lettuce water: Take leaf lettuce and boil in water, drink 4 ozs. every hour. Echinacea (homeopathic): For viral infections in blood and lymph.
Vision, dimness		Linden flower, carrot juice A tea combination of parsley leaves, parsley root, marshmallow root, and uva ursi leaves.
Vision, objects look distorted in size		Nutmeg: Use ¼ tsp. in 6 ozs. of hot water.
Vitality, low	B-complex, B_1, C, E, pantothenic acid	
Vitamin C replacement		Alfalfa seed Cranberry juice: Frequently recommended for people whose body is not utilizing vitamin C properly. The best time to drink it is early afternoon. Make sure you drink cranberry juice and not cranapple or other mixes.

HEALTH ISSUE	REMEDIES

	Vitamins/ Minerals	Spices/Herbs/ Kitchen Aids
Voice, hoarse (see also Hoarseness; Laryngitis)		Mullein leaf tea: Use as needed.
Voice box gives out	Sulfur	
Vomiting of food (chronic)		Cinnamon and nutmeg also help relieve nausea. Dill seed: Use ½ tsp. in water or chew it. Vinegar: In case of severe vomiting, moisten a cloth with warm vinegar and apply over abdomen.
Walking, cannot on uneven ground		Tiger lily (*Lilium tigrinum*) (homeopathic)
Warts	A, E, silicon	Castor oil: Apply a few drops to wart and bandage tightly. Repeat 2 or 3 times daily until wart disappears. Dandelion juice or milkweed juice: Apply topically. Dulcamara (homeopathic): Use for warts on hands and face. Fenugreek seed: Soak seed in water until it makes a mucilage-like ointment. Apply to the wart and let dry. Use once daily until the wart disappears. Lemon peel: For calluses, corns, or warts. Put the lemon peel (white side down) on the afflicted area overnight. *Thuja occidentalis* (homeopathic)

HEALTH ISSUE   REMEDIES

	Vitamins/ Minerals	Spices/Herbs/ Kitchen Aids
Warts (cont.)		Willow leaf (fresh): Squeeze the juice on the wart.
Warts, plantar (foot)		Chalk: Oil a piece of cloth, grate regular chalk over the oiled area and apply overnight. Do this for 14 days.
Water retention	Potassium	Banana is a good potassium fruit. If taken in moderation, will balance excess water in the system. Fennel, watermelon seed tea, parsley tea Nettle (2 parts), uva ursi (1 part): Mix, make tea, and drink 4 cups daily to eliminate excess water from the cells. Woodruff tea: 3 cups daily.
Weak, digestion		Cashew nut (*Anacardium occidentale*)
Weak, joints		Ginger tea
Weak, ligaments	Potassium, E, C	
Weak, memory		Club moss
Weak, muscles		Dried apples peelings made into tea strengthen muscles and improve other kinds of weakness. Lady's mantle (*Alchemilla vulgaris*)
Weak, stomach		Rosemary, sorrel

HEALTH ISSUE	REMEDIES	
	Vitamins/ Minerals	Spices/Herbs/ Kitchen Aids
Weakness, in the elderly and debilitated		Arrowroot: It is easily digested, creating no gastric upset. Yarrow tea: Drink 2 cups daily.
Weak-willed		Sesame seeds: They are a complete amino acid supplier and make strong-willed people. They supply osmium, a trace mineral.
Weight loss (see Antifat; Obesity; Overweight; Reducing)		
Whooping cough	B₆	Red clover Rub onion juice into soles of feet or into the back. Or ginger tea or 1 tbl. thyme, boil in 1 cup water for 20 minutes, strain, add honey, take 1 tsp. every hour.
Wickedness		Cashew nut (*Anacardium occidentale*)
Winding motion of body	Magnesium	
Without joy	Sulfur	
Women, with biting dispositions		Cramp bark
Women's ailments (repeated)	Sulfur	
Worms (see also Parasites; Vermifuge)	Calcium (when worms are repeated)	Birch leaves or bark; Blue cohosh Figs: Eat 3 or 4 figs twice daily.

HEALTH ISSUE	REMEDIES	
	Vitamins/ Minerals	Spices/Herbs/ Kitchen Aids
Worms (cont.)		Garlic: Cut 3 cloves, boil in 8 ozs. of milk for 5 minutes, let cool so you can drink it. Do this before going to sleep for 10 days in a row.
		Pomegranate: As juice or eaten raw. Helps keep worms out of system.
		Pumpkin seeds: Eat ½ cup pumpkin seeds a day, especially before a meal on an empty stomach. Worms are stripped from their protective skins by pumpkin seeds.
		White figs are useful for de-worming. Figs and fig juice paralyze any worm, even the tapeworm, pin-worm, and roundworm.
Worry, in elderly		Larkspur tea: 1 tsp. to 1 cup of boiling water. Drink 1 cup 4 times daily.
Wrinkles		Cowslip oil Hellebore: for forehead Violet root: for hands and feet White hellebore tea: Wash in it; also for hands and feet

Chapter Sixteen

❋

HERBS AND FORMULAS

Any herb types referred to in previous chapters are included here. The herbs are categorized for your convenience, and healing oil and tincture recipes are also included.

Categorizing Herbs

We are accustomed to categorizing our lives and also our environments. Reluctantly, I do so with herbs—the medicine of the ages, the medicine of God's drugstore.

This outline is only a small portion of herbs in your vicinity. By walking through the meadows you will easily find the iron herbs, the magnesium herbs, and so on.

Calcium Herbs   Caraway seeds, Chamomile, Chives, Cleavers, Coltsfoot, Dandelion, Dill, Horsetail, Pimpernel, Tormentil root

Chlorine Herbs   Fennel, Goldenseal, Myrrh, Nettle, Plantain, Uva Ursi, Watercress, Wintergreen

Copper Herbs	Dandelion, Devil's Bit, Liverwort, Salep, Sheep Sorrel
Fluorine Herbs	Cornsilk, Dill, Horsetail, Oats, Plantain, Thyme, Watercress
Iodine Herbs	Algae, Dulse, Iceland Moss, Irish Moss, Kelp, Mustard, Nettle, Parsley, Sea Wrack
Iron Herbs	Burdock, Dandelion, Huckleberry Leaves, Irish Moss, Meadowsweet, Sheep Sorrel, Silverweed, Stinging Nettle, Strawberry Leaves, Yellow Dock
Magnesium Herbs	Broom Tops, Carrot Leaves, Devil's Bit, Meadowsweet, Mullein Leaves, Nettle, Primrose, Walnut Leaves
Manganese Herbs	Burdock, Kelp, Sheep Sorrel, Strawberry Leaves, Wintergreen, Yellow Dock
Nickel Herbs	Algae, Bladderwrack, Kelp, Liverwort
Phosphorus Herbs	Calamus, Chickweed, Dill, Licorice Root, Marigold Flowers, Rhubarb, Sorrel, Watercress
Potassium Herbs	American Centaury, Carrot Leaves, Comfrey, Couch Grass, Mullein, Oak Bark, Plantain Leaves, Primrose Flowers, Summer Savory, Walnut Leaves, Yarrow
Silicon Herbs	Chickweed, Cornsilk, Flaxseed, Horsetail, Lamb's-quarters, Oat Straw, Red Raspberry Leaves, Sunflower Seeds
Sodium Herbs	Apple Tree Bark, Celery Seed, Cleavers, Dill, Fennel Seed, Huckleberry Leaves, Meadowsweet, Mistletoe, Stinging Nettle
Sulfur Herbs	Coltsfoot, Eyebright, Fennel, Meadowsweet, Mullein, Pimpernel, Plantain Leaves, Scouring Rush, Shepherd's Purse, Stinging Nettle, Watercress
Zinc Herbs	Horsetail, Paprika, Shepherd's Purse

Healing Oils and Tinctures

HEALING OIL RECIPE

Take 2 handfuls of fresh herbs or 1 handful of dried herbs. Cover with olive oil. Let stand in a warm place for 14 days, stirring once in a while. After 14 days, simmer for 15 minutes and strain. Squeeze the last drop of oil out of the mixture. Again put 2 handfuls of fresh herbs or 1 handful of dried herbs in the leftover oil and, placing it in a warm place, repeat the procedure. After 14 days, bring it to a boil and simmer it again for 15 minutes. Strain and squeeze out the last drop of oil. There is not much left; however, the oil is mighty potent, and you need only a few drops.

Use the above recipe for any of the following oils:

Calendula Oil	Good for boils and everything that does not want to heal.
Chamomile Oil	Good for cramplike pains.
Dill Oil	Can be rubbed on all aching parts of body.
Juniper Oil	Good for cramps in legs, pain in hips, and paralysis.
Lily Oil	Helps spasms, tendons, wrinkles, and scars.
Peppermint Oil	Helps frozen fingers or ears. Good for scars or calluses.

TINCTURE RECIPE

Take any herb, preferably fresh, and place in a jar that has a tight-fitting lid. Cover with 80 proof alcohol (not rubbing alcohol) and let it sit in a warm place for 10 to 14 days, stirring once in a while. After 14 days, strain and fill into bottle. Use only small amounts, for it is potent.

ABOUT THE AUTHOR

The late **Hanna Kroeger** was the daughter of German missionaries. She studied nursing at the University of Freiburg, Germany, and worked in a hospital for natural healing under Professor Brauchle. In 1953, she and her family came to America.

After coming to the United States, Hanna took advantage of the education offered by the American systems, ranging from Amerindian herbology to massage. She had a Doctorate of Metaphysics (MsD), and was an ordained minister in the Universal Church of the Masters, a church well known for its work in contact and spiritual healing. Besides teaching and lecturing, she ran a health food store in Colorado, and for years owned and operated a health resort, the Peaceful Meadow Retreat, where she saw her knowledge of nutrition used with exciting results.

For information on the herbs and home remedies in this book, please call Hanna's Herb Shop at 800-206-6722.

We hope you enjoyed this Hay House book.
If you would like to receive a free catalog featuring
additional Hay House books and products,
or if you would like information about
the Hay Foundation, please write to:

Hay House, Inc.
P.O. Box 5100
Carlsbad, CA 92018-5100

(760) 431-7695 or (800) 654-5126
(760) 431-6948 (fax) or (800) 650-5115 (fax)

Please visit the Hay House Website at:
www.hayhouse.com